MW01533468

Regional Anesthesia
UPDATES
Fast-Track Updates for Busy Clinicians

2025 EDITION

Authors

Admir Hadzic, MD, PhD
Catherine Vandepitte, MD, PhD

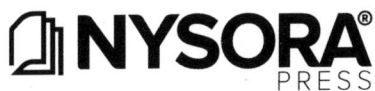

NYSORA® PRESS

Publishing Division of NYSORA, Inc
2585 Broadway, suite 183, New York, NY10025
info@nysora.com, www.nysora.com

Contributors: NYSORA Educational Board

- Stien Beyens, Msc | NYSORA, Leuven, Belgium
- Jirka Cops, PhD | NYSORA, Leuven, Belgium
- Darren Jacobs, Msc | NYSORA, Leuven, Belgium
- Jill Vanhaeren, Msc | NYSORA, Leuven, Belgium
- Dr. Preeti Anand, MD | Department of Anesthesiology, Albert Einstein College of Medicine, New York City, New York, USA
- Dr. Pietro Balagna, MD | Department of Translational Medicine, University of Eastern Piedmont, Novara, Italy | Department of Anesthesiology, St-Luc Hospital, UCLouvain, Brussels, Belgium
- Dr. Angela Lucia Balocco, MD | Department of Anesthesiology, UZ Leuven, Leuven, Belgium | Faculty of Medicine and Life Sciences, Hasselt University, Hasselt, Belgium
- Dr. Vipin Bansal, MD | Department of anesthesiology, Emory University School of Medicine, Atlanta, Georgia, USA | Department of anesthesiology and pain medicine, Children's Healthcare of Atlanta, Atlanta, Georgia, USA
- Dr. Amy Belba, MD | Department of Anesthesiology and Intensive Care, Ziekenhuis Oost-Limburg, Genk, Belgium | Department of Anesthesiology and Pain Medicine, Maastricht University Medical Center+, Maastricht, The Netherlands | Faculty of Medicine and Life Sciences, Hasselt University, Hasselt, Belgium
- Dr. Dominique Chang, MD | Department of Anesthesiology, Albert Einstein College of Medicine, New York City, New York, USA
- Dr. Matthew Colontonio, MD | Department of Anesthesiology and Perioperative Medicine, Mayo Clinic, Jacksonville, Florida, USA
- Dr. Olivier De Fré, MD | Department of Anesthesiology, AZHerentals, Herentals, Belgium
- Dr. Anthony Deman, MD | Department of Anesthesiology and Intensive Care, Ziekenhuis Oost-Limburg, Genk, Belgium
- Dr. Dimitri Dylst, MD | Department of Anesthesiology and Intensive Care, Ziekenhuis Oost-Limburg, Genk, Belgium
- Dr. Christian Horazeck, MD, D.ABA | Department of Anesthesiology and Acute Pain Management, Baylor Scott & White, Temple, Texas, USA
- Dr. Jona Houthuys, MD | Department of Anesthesiology and Intensive Care, Ziekenhuis Oost-Limburg, Genk, Belgium
- Dr. Jerry Jones, MD | Department of Anesthesiology, College of Medicine, UTHSC, Memphis, Tennessee, USA
- Dr. Ivan Keser, MD | Department of Anesthesiology, General Hospital "Prim.dr. Abdullah Nakaš" Sarajevo, Bosnia and Herzegovina
- Dr. Fadi Kadourra, MD | Department of Pain Medicine, Cleveland Clinic, Abu Dhabi, United Arab Emirates
- Dr. Samantha Kransingh, MD | Acute Pain Service Lead, Te Whatu Ora South Canterbury, New Zealand
- Dr. Queenayda Kroon, MD, FIPP | Department of Anesthesiology, ZorgSaam, Terneuzen, Zeeland, The Netherlands
- Dr. Kwesi Kwofie, MD, FRCPC | Department of Anesthesia, Pain Management & Perioperative Medicine, Faculty of Medicine, Dalhousie University, Halifax, Canada
- Dr. Isabelle Lenders, MD | Department of Anesthesiology and Intensive Care, Ziekenhuis Oost-Limburg, Genk, Belgium
- Dr. Ana Lopez Gutiérrez, MD, PhD | Department of Anesthesiology and Intensive Care, Ziekenhuis Oost-Limburg, Genk, Belgium
- Dr. Sofie Louage, MD | Department of Anesthesiology, AZ Glorieux, Ronse, Belgium
- Dr. Leander Mancel, MD | Department of Anesthesiology and Intensive Care, Ziekenhuis Oost-Limburg, Genk, Belgium
- Dr. Daniela Nieuwveld, MD| Department of Anesthesiology, Hospital del Mar, Barcelona, Spain
- Dr. Simon Njuguna, MD, FIPP, DESAIC | Department of Anesthesiology, ASZ Aalst, Belgium
- Dr. Chang Park, MD | Department of Anesthesiology, Icahn School of Medicine at Mount Sinai, New York, USA
- Dr. Laurens Peene, MD | Department of Anesthesiology and Intensive Care, Ziekenhuis Oost-Limburg, Genk, Belgium
- Dr. Florence Polfliet, MD | Department of Anesthesiology and Intensive Care, Ziekenhuis Oost-Limburg, Genk, Belgium
- Dr. Fréderic Polus, MD | Department of Anesthesiology, Noorderhart Mariaziekenhuis, Pelt, Belgium
- Dr. Amar Salti, MD | Cleveland Clinic, Abu Dhabi, UAE
- Dr. Aysu Salviz, MD, ESRA-DRA | Department of Anesthesiology, Washington University, St. Louis, Missouri, USA
- Dr. Sarah Siba, MD | Department of Anesthesiology and Intensive Care, Ziekenhuis Oost-Limburg, Genk, Belgium
- Victor Coll Sijercic, BSc | Faculty of Osteopathic Medicine, Noorda College of Osteopathic Medicine, Utah, USA
- Dr. Walter Staelens, MD| Department of Anesthesiology and Intensive care, Ziekenhuis Oost-Limburg, Genk, Belgium
- Dr. Imré Van Herreweghe, MD | Department of Anesthesiology and Intensive Care, Ziekenhuis Oost-Limburg, Genk, Belgium
- Dr. Astrid Van Lantschoot, MD | Department of Anesthesiology and Intensive Care, Ziekenhuis Oost-Limburg, Genk, Belgium
- Dr. Stefanie Vanhoenacker, MD | Department of Anesthesiology, St-Jozefskliniek, Izegem, Belgium
- Dr. Thibaut Vanneste, MD | Department of Anesthesiology and Intensive Care, Ziekenhuis Oost-Limburg, Genk, Belgium
- Dr. Arnaud Weynants, MD | Department of Anesthesiology and Intensive Care, Ziekenhuis Oost-Limburg, Genk, Belgium

▉ Introduction

In an era of increasing demands on clinicians-balancing patient care, administrative duties, and the ongoing need for professional development-keeping up with the latest advancements in regional anesthesia has become an ever-greater challenge. New techniques, pharmacological advancements, and clinical guidelines are emerging at a rapid pace, while the decline of dedicated journals has left a void in readily accessible, peer-reviewed resources.

Recognizing this need, *NYSORA's Regional Anesthesia Updates 2025* was created to deliver concise, actionable insights tailored for the busy practitioner, comprising carefully selected the most important literature updates from the past 12 months or so. This book is the product of NYSORA's international Educational Board, which comprises world-renowned scholars, educators, and highly skilled clinicians. Every chapter undergoes a rigorous two-step peer-review process, blending the expertise of NYSORA's fellows, collaborators, and external reviewers. This ensures each update is not only accurate and clinically relevant but also directly applicable to everyday practice.

Structured for efficiency, the updates in this book distill the most important developments in regional anesthesia into 10-minute reads or less. Each topic highlights key findings from the latest clinical trials, innovations, and comparative studies without burdening the reader with excessive details on methodology or analytics. Instead, the focus is on practical, evidence-based insights designed to enhance clinical decision-making and patient outcomes.

NYSORA's Regional Anesthesia Updates 2025 also reflect the contributions of its global network of collaborators, whose work ensures the content remains cutting-edge and comprehensive. The book is organized into relevance-based sections for easy navigation, with space provided for personal notes to adapt the material to individual practice needs.

Whether you are a seasoned anesthesiologist or a trainee, this book serves as an indispensable resource to keep you at the forefront of regional anesthesia. With NYSORA's decades of expertise and the collective wisdom of its international Educational Board, this volume is more than a compilation of updates-it's a tool to inspire better patient care and continuous professional growth.

Drs Hadzic and Vandepitte & NYSORA Team

Dedication

To the practitioners whose skill and dedication bring the science of regional anesthesia to life, improving patient outcomes every day.

To the students and trainees who represent the future of this field, inspiring us with their curiosity, determination, and drive for excellence.

And to the patients whose trust motivates us to continually advance the practice of regional anesthesia and analgesia, ensuring safer, more effective, and compassionate care.

This book is for you-may it serve as a resource, a guide, and a source of inspiration in your journey.

Acknowledgments

Thank YOU:

To the extraordinary team behind NYSORA, whose dedication and expertise have made this book a reality.

To the *NYSORA Scientific Team*, whose unwavering commitment to excellence ensures the accuracy, relevance, and impact of every update.

To the *NYSORA Educational Board*, our global network of scholars, educators, and clinicians, for their insightful contributions and rigorous peer reviews.

To the *NYSORA Designers*, whose creativity transforms complex knowledge into visually engaging and accessible formats, bringing our mission to life.

And to every collaborator, fellow, and member of NYSORA community-thank you for your passion, innovation, and tireless work in advancing the field of regional anesthesia.

This book is a testament to your brilliance and dedication to improving patient care worldwide.

Copyright 2024 by Nysora, Inc. All rights reserved. No part of this publication can be reproduced or distributed in any form or by any means, or stored in a database or retrieval system, without the prior written permission of the publisher.

Notice / Disclaimer

The information contained in *Regional Anesthesia Updates 2025* is intended to serve as a guide for practicing clinicians in the field of anesthesiology, pain medicine, and perioperative care. NYSORA Press and its contributors have made every effort to ensure the accuracy, completeness, and relevance of the content presented. However, medical knowledge is continually evolving, and new research or clinical guidelines may emerge after the publication of this book.

NYSORA Press and NYSORA Inc. do not assume any liability or responsibility for any errors, omissions, or potential consequences arising from using the information provided. The clinical recommendations, techniques, and drug dosages presented in this text should be interpreted and applied by qualified healthcare professionals in conjunction with their clinical judgment, institutional protocols, and current best practices.

Ultimately, the responsibility for patient care lies with the attending healthcare professional, and any application of the information provided in this text must be tailored to each patient's specific circumstances.

NYSORA Press and NYSORA Inc. expressly disclaim any liability for adverse outcomes, including but not limited to injury, illness, or death, that may result from the application or interpretation of the content within *Regional Anesthesia Updates 2025*.

By utilizing this book, readers acknowledge and accept that the responsibility for safe and effective patient care rests with the clinician's professional judgment and the proper application of current medical standards and practices.

Errata: While every effort has been made to ensure the accuracy and quality of this book, errors or areas for improvement may still exist. If you identify any inaccuracies or have suggestions for enhancing the content or visuals, please send your feedback to info@nysora.com. We value your input and may acknowledge contributions as appropriate. Thank you for supporting our commitment to continuous improvement.

Library of Congress Identification

Authors: Admir Hadzic, MD, PhD | Catherine Vandepitte, MD, PhD

Title: Regional Anesthesia Updates
Subtitle: Fast-Track Updates for Busy Clinicians
2025 Edition

Identifiers:
Library of Congress Control Number: 2024926444
ISBN: 979-8-9920578-3-6

Table of Contents

Innovations in block techniques and pain management

Regional anesthesia for pediatric and geriatric patients

Safety and risk management

Special considerations in neuraxial anesthesia

Multimodal pain management and outcomes

Emerging insights and comparisons of techniques

Foundations and innovations in regional anesthesia

Optimized strategies for single-shot and continuous blocks

01

Why this topic is important

Regional anesthesia has revolutionized perioperative pain management, providing effective analgesia while minimizing reliance on opioids. With advancements in ultrasound technology, regional techniques have expanded significantly, enabling precise and effective block administration. As the field evolves, optimizing single-shot and continuous peripheral nerve blocks (CPNBs) has become essential to enhance outcomes, minimize complications, and maximize patient satisfaction. Based on a review by Johnstone et al. in *Current Opinion in Anesthesiology (2024)*, this update consolidates recent findings to provide insights into best practices, technological advancements, and future directions in regional anesthesia.

Objectives of this update

- Highlight recent advancements in single-shot and continuous peripheral nerve block techniques.

- Explore strategies for enhancing block efficacy, safety, and patient outcomes.

- Address educational and technological innovations shaping the future of regional anesthesia.

What is new

This review offers fresh perspectives, including:

- Advances in anatomy and pharmacology for safer and more effective block placement.

- Technological innovations like artificial intelligence (AI) and simulation to improve block accuracy and training.

- Education-focused strategies, such as standardized "Plan A" blocks, for enhancing skills among general anesthesiologists.

Pain management

- Role of regional anesthesia in acute and chronic pain:

  ○ Ultrasound-guided regional anesthesia (UGRA) effectively manages acute pain, reducing the need for systemic opioids.

  ○ However, its role in chronic pain and long-term risk modification remains under investigation.

- Adjuncts for prolonged efficacy:

  ○ Dexamethasone, administered intravenously or perineurally, extends block duration, with a plateau effect observed at 4 mg perineurally and 8 mg intravenously.

  ○ Liposomal bupivacaine offers sustained analgesia in approved indications but lacks robust evidence to support its superiority over standard long-acting anesthetics in some off-label indications.

Conduct and efficacy of regional anesthesia

- Technical expertise:

  ○ Optimal outcomes require precise needle placement guided by ultrasound imaging and an understanding of nerve anatomy.

  ○ Studies suggest targeting the space between the innermost circumneural fascial layer and the outer epineurium to maximize efficacy and minimize injury risks.

- Innovations in dose minimization:

  ○ Research has refined the minimum effective volumes for local anesthetics, ensuring efficacy while reducing complications. For example, 2.5 mL of 0.5% bupivacaine per nerve may be sufficient to achieve surgical anesthesia during axillary brachial plexus blocks.

- Safe block practices:

  ○ Initiatives like "Prep, Stop, Block" emphasize safety, reducing the incidence of wrong-site nerve blocks through standardized operating procedures.

Education and training

- "Plan A" blocks:

  ○ Standardized blocks, such as "Plan A," focus on high-value, versatile techniques for training general anesthesiologists. These blocks address common surgical and pain indications, ensuring widespread applicability.

- Simulation-based mastery learning:

  ○ Simulation training accelerates skill acquisition by providing safe, hands-on practice with immediate feedback. Advances include augmented reality tools like NeedleTrainer for needle guidance and positioning.

- International consensus:

  ○ Collaboration between organizations like ASRA and ESRA has standardized block nomenclature and ultrasound landmarks, enhancing global consistency in training and research.

Technological innovations

- Artificial intelligence:

  ○ AI tools, such as ScanNav, enhance ultrasound-guided block accuracy by providing real-time anatomical overlays, boosting confidence and success rates among novice practitioners.

- Needle tracking:

  ○ Systems like Onvision improve needle tip visualization, reducing complications and improving procedural safety.

- Ultrasound advancements:

  ○ Innovations such as ultrasonic needle technology and fiber-optic tracking systems improve visibility and accuracy, though clinical studies remain limited.

Limitations

- Research gaps:
    - Limited evidence exists for the long-term benefits of certain technologies, such as AI-assisted ultrasound and liposomal bupivacaine.

- Training variability:
    - Access to high-fidelity simulations and advanced training tools may be restricted to larger academic centers.

Key takeaways

☑ Optimized regional anesthesia combines advanced techniques, pharmacology, and technology to deliver superior analgesia and safety.

☑ Standardized training strategies, such as "Plan A" blocks, ensure skill acquisition across diverse clinical settings.

☑ Technological innovations, including AI and needle tracking, hold promise for improving block accuracy and reducing complications.

☑ Continued research and collaboration are essential to refine practices and expand the accessibility of regional anesthesia.

Additional recommended reading

1. Johnstone D, Taylor A, Ferry J. Optimizing peripheral regional anesthesia: Strategies for single-shot and continuous blocks. *Curr Opin Anesthesiol.* 2024;37:541-546.

2. Zufferey PJ, Chaux R, Lachaud PA, et al. Dose-response relationships of intravenous and perineural dexamethasone as adjuvants to peripheral nerve blocks: A systematic review and model-based network meta-analysis. *Br J Anaesth.* 2024;132:1122-1132.

3. Bowness JS, Macfarlane AJR, Burckett-St Laurent D, et al. Evaluation of the impact of assistive artificial intelligence on ultrasound scanning for regional anesthesia. *Br J Anaesth.* 2023;130:226-233.

Risk of neurological injury following peripheral nerve blocks and the role of ultrasound guidance

02

Why this topic is important

Peripheral nerve blocks (PNBs) are key to modern regional anesthesia, offering benefits like improved analgesia, reduced opioid use, and faster recovery. Despite their advantages, neurological complications, such as post-block neurological dysfunction (PBND), remain a concern. Although PBND is rare, its potential to cause sensorimotor deficits lasting beyond the block's expected duration poses risks for patients.

Seddon's classification of nerve injuries

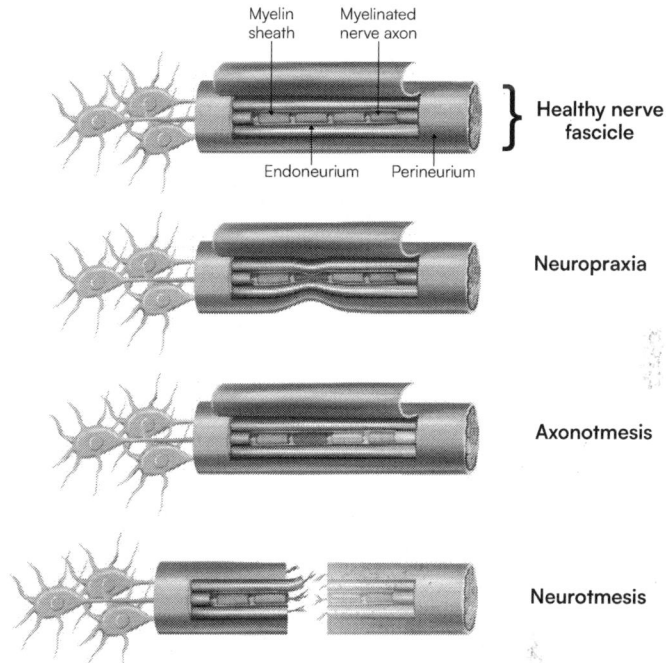

Fig-1. Seddon initially proposed the classification of peripheral nerve injury (PNI), which categorizes injuries based on the severity of damage. These classifications help predict the prognosis and guide clinical management. Image taken from NYSORA LMS. https://nysoralms.com/

With ultrasound (US) guidance becoming the standard for PNBs, its potential to reduce neurological complications warrants investigation. This review consolidates current data on PBND incidence, time-dependent recovery, and the protective role of US guidance.

Objectives of this update

- To estimate the pooled incidence of PBND following PNBs over various timeframes.

- To compare the incidence of PBND between PNBs performed with and without US guidance.

- To identify blocks with a higher risk of neurological complications and suggest measures to minimize risks.

What is new

This review by Lemke et al. 2024 provides comprehensive data from 92 studies - encompassing a total of 1,553,000 patients - assessing PBND incidence at multiple time points. It confirms that PBND rates decrease over time and highlights the role of US guidance in reducing risks, particularly for high-risk blocks like interscalene and axillary brachial plexus blocks.

Key findings

Incidence of PBND

- Time-dependent trends:

  - PBND incidence was approximately 1% at 2 weeks (9 per 1,000 blocks), reducing to 0.03% at 1 year (0.3 per 1,000 blocks).

  - Most cases are resolved within 2 weeks, emphasizing the transient nature of many neurological injuries.

- Block-specific risks:

  - Interscalene blocks showed the highest PBND incidence at 2 weeks (2.2%) compared to other blocks.

  - Lower extremity blocks (e.g., femoral, popliteal) had significantly lower PBND rates, potentially due to differences in nerve architecture and connective tissue density.

PNBD incidence decline. Table adapted from Lemke et al. 2024[1]

Time point	Overall PBND incidence (per 1000 blocks)	With US guidance (per 1000 blocks)	Without US guidance (per 1000 blocks)
< 2 weeks	9	12	8
3-6 weeks	4	3	6
7 weeks-5 months	3	3	3
6 months-1 year	1	0.04	1
> 1 year	0.3	0.1	0.8

Impact of ultrasound guidance

- Reduced PBND incidence:

  - PNBs performed with US guidance had lower pooled PBND rates than non-US techniques.

  - For interscalene blocks, US guidance halved the incidence of PBND at 2 weeks (1.1% with US vs. 3.2% without US (11 per 1,000 blocks vs. 32 per 1,000 blocks).

  - Differences were less pronounced for lower extremity blocks, which inherently carry lower risks of nerve injury.

- Technical advantages of US guidance:

- Improved visualization reduces the need for multiple needle passes and minimizes the risk of intraneural injections.

- Enables precise delivery of local anesthetic, potentially reducing mechanical or ischemic nerve injuries.

Clinical implications

Identifying and mitigating risks

- High-risk blocks: Interscalene and axillary brachial plexus blocks require cautious technique and preferential use of US guidance.

- Timing of recovery: Most PBND cases resolve within weeks, but persistent cases beyond 6 months necessitate further evaluation.

Optimizing safety with ultrasound guidance

- US guidance enhances safety for PNBs, particularly for blocks involving compact nerve structures.

- Encouraging its use universally can lower PBND rates and improve patient outcomes.

Patient counseling and follow-up

- Patients should be informed of the low but present risk of PBND, including expected recovery timelines.

- Standardized follow-up protocols are essential to detect and address persistent neurological deficits promptly.

Limitations

- Limited data for intermediate (7 weeks-5 months) and long-term (> 1 year) PBND outcomes.

- Variability in study designs and definitions of PBND complicates direct comparisons.

Key takeaways

☑ PBND following PNBs is rare and often transient, with the incidence decreasing over time.

☑ Ultrasound guidance reduces PBND rates, especially for high-risk blocks like interscalene.

☑ Most cases resolve within 2 weeks; persistent symptoms should prompt evaluation.

☑ Broader adoption of US guidance and standardized reporting can enhance safety and outcomes.

Additional recommended reading

1. Lemke E, Johnston DF, Behrens MB, et al. Neurological injury following peripheral nerve blocks: A narrative review of estimates of risks and the influence of ultrasound guidance. *Reg Anesth Pain Med.* 2024;49:122-132.

2. Brull R, Hadzic A, Reina MA, et al. Pathophysiology and etiology of nerve injury following peripheral nerve blockade. *Reg Anesth Pain Med.* 2015;40:479-90.

3. Neal JM, Barrington MJ, Brull R, et al. The second ASRA practice advisory on neurologic complications associated with regional anesthesia and pain medicine: Executive summary. *Reg Anesth Pain Med.* 2015;40:401-30.

Combined dexamethasone and dexmedetomidine as adjuncts to peripheral nerve blocks

03

Why this topic is important

Peripheral nerve blocks (PNBs) provide effective pain relief and minimize opioid use. The duration of analgesia remains a key challenge, leading to an increased interest in adjuncts like dexamethasone and dexmedetomidine. Both agents have demonstrated block-prolonging effects individually, but their combined impact needs to be clarified. A recent systematic review by Maagaard et al. 2024 evaluates the effects of combining dexamethasone and dexmedetomidine on analgesic duration and other outcomes, offering valuable insights for optimizing regional anesthesia protocols.

Objectives of this update

- To assess the impact of combined dexamethasone and dexmedetomidine on analgesic duration in PNBs.

- To evaluate its effects on motor and sensory block duration, opioid consumption, and adverse events.

- To provide evidence-based guidance on the utility of this combination in clinical practice.

What is new

This review by Magaard et al. 2024 is the first systematic review and meta-analysis to analyze the combined use of dexamethasone and dexmedetomidine as adjuncts in PNBs. It draws data from 9 randomized controlled trials (RCTs) and offers robust conclusions through trial sequential analysis (TSA).

Key findings

Duration of analgesia

1. Compared to placebo:

   - The combination extended the analgesic duration by 460 minutes.

   - TSA confirmed sufficient evidence for at least a 33% increase in block duration over placebo.

2. Compared to dexamethasone alone:

   - No significant difference in analgesic duration.

   - TSA showed that the required sample size was achieved, confirming no substantial additive effect over dexamethasone alone.

3. Compared to dexmedetomidine alone:

   - The combination significantly increased analgesic duration by 388 minutes.

Other outcomes

1. Motor block duration:

   - Extended significantly compared to placebo.

   - Similar duration when compared with dexamethasone or dexmedetomidine alone.

2. Sensory block duration:

   - Data were inconsistent, but trends favored the combination over dexmedetomidine and showed equivalence to dexamethasone.

3. Opioid consumption (24 hours):

   - It is likely reduced with the combination versus placebo.

   - There was no significant reduction compared to dexamethasone or dexmedetomidine alone.

4. Adverse events:

   - The combination showed similar rates of adverse events as placebo, dexamethasone, or dexmedetomidine, but the evidence was uncertain due to small sample sizes.

Clinical implications

Use of the combination

- The combination of dexamethasone and dexmedetomidine significantly prolongs analgesic duration compared to dexmedetomidine alone or placebo.

- Its lack of additive benefit over dexamethasone alone suggests limited utility when dexamethasone is already being used.

Practical recommendations

- Dexamethasone alone remains a strong choice for prolonging block duration, given its similar efficacy and established safety profile.

- The combination may be considered when both agents' mechanisms are required, such as when longer motor or sensory block durations are beneficial.

Limitations

- There is a high risk of bias in most included trials.

- Heterogeneity in definitions of block duration (e.g., time to first pain vs. first analgesic request).

Key takeaways

- ☑ Combined dexamethasone and dexmedetomidine extend analgesic duration compared to placebo or dexmedetomidine alone but show no significant benefit over dexamethasone alone.

- ☑ Use dexamethasone as the primary adjunct for PNBs when the goal is analgesic prolongation.

- ☑ The combination may be reserved for specific cases requiring enhanced block duration.

Additional recommended reading

1. Maagaard M, Andersen JH, Jaeger P, et al. Effects of combined dexamethasone and dexmedetomidine as adjuncts to peripheral nerve blocks: A systematic review with meta-analysis and trial sequential analysis. *Reg Anesth Pain Med.* 2024;49:1-10.

2. Pehora C, Pearson AM, Kaushal A, et al. Dexamethasone as an adjuvant to peripheral nerve block. *Cochrane Database Syst Rev.* 2017;11:CD011770.

3. Abdallah FW, Dwyer T, Chan VWS, et al. IV and perineural dexmedetomidine similarly prolong the duration of analgesia after interscalene brachial plexus block: A randomized trial. *Anesthesiology.* 2016;124:683-95.

Peripheral nerve microanatomy and adipose compartments to enhance block success

04

Why this topic is important

Peripheral nerve blocks (PNBs) are a cornerstone of regional anesthesia, offering pain relief and reduced opioid consumption. However, variability in block success, duration, and potential complications suggests gaps in our understanding of the mechanisms involved. Traditional models have emphasized the epineurium and perineurium as critical structures but have overlooked the role of perineural adipose compartments and collagen fibers.

A recent review by Mcleod et al. (RAPM, 2024) integrates new microanatomical findings and micro-ultrasound data, shedding light on how adipose tissue and fascia influence local anesthetic (LA) spread, block efficacy, and needle placement techniques.

Objectives of this update

- To examine how adipose compartments and collagen fiber layers impact nerve block outcomes.

- To challenge traditional nerve anatomy paradigms with emerging microanatomical evidence.

- To propose practical implications for enhancing block success and safety.

What is new

The review by Mcleod et al. 2024 reveals that adipose compartments, surrounded by interlaced collagen fibers, play a crucial role in determining LA distribution, injection pressure, and block quality. These findings advocate for refined needle placement techniques and advanced imaging to optimize outcomes.

Key findings

Adipose tissue compartments and their role in nerve blocks

1. Compartmentalization:

   ○ Nerves are surrounded by non-communicating adipose tissue compartments encased in circumneurium and epineurium.

   ○ These compartments restrict LA spread, influencing block density and duration.

2. Injection dynamics:

   ○ LA injected into these compartments remains confined unless the needle tip moves, causing variability in spread and efficacy.

   ○ Collagen fibers within the compartments impede LA movement, altering onset and block quality.

3. Protective function:

   ○ Adipose tissue cushions nerves, reducing mechanical trauma and supporting vascular structures.

Microanatomical and micro-ultrasound insights

1. High-definition imaging:

   ○ Ultra-high-resolution micro-ultrasound (> 30 MHz) has revealed intricate adipose tissue arrangements previously undetectable with standard ultrasound.

   ○ These findings challenge assumptions about needle placement accuracy and the predictability of LA spread.

2. Intraneural injections:

   ○ Intraneural adipose tissue allows LA to spread without damaging fascicles if injected correctly.

   ○ Misinterpreting spread patterns on clinical ultrasound may lead to incorrect assessments of needle location.

3. Injection pressure:

   • Due to varying tissue resistance, pressure measurements alone are unreliable for determining needle-tip location.

Clinical implications

Enhancing block success

• Optimizing needle placement:

   ○ Targeting subcircumneural adipose layers may improve LA delivery to nerve bundles, enhancing block efficacy.

   ○ Gentle needle apposition to the epineurium, verified by slight nerve displacement, is recommended.

• Refining injection techniques:

   ○ A slow, controlled injection allows LA to disperse within adipose compartments without exceeding pressure thresholds.

Improving safety

• Mitigating complications:

   ○ Recognizing the protective role of adipose tissue can guide safer intraneural injection practices.

   ○ Standard ultrasound's inability to distinguish fascicular boundaries highlights the need for improved imaging tools.

Practical considerations

• Current ultrasound equipment may not resolve microanatomical features critical for precise needle placement.

• Combining imaging, anatomical knowledge, and electrical nerve stimulation is crucial for continuous PNBs.

Limitations and future directions

Study limitations

- Most findings are based on cadaveric and animal models, limiting direct clinical application.
- Standard ultrasound resolution is insufficient for visualizing adipose tissue compartments in vivo.

Recommendations for future research

- Explore clinical applications of micro-ultrasound to improve needle placement accuracy.
- Investigate the impact of adipose tissue variability on LA pharmacodynamics and patient outcomes.
- Develop standardized protocols for targeting adipose compartments in PNBs.

Key takeaways

☑ Adipose compartments and collagen fibers influence LA spread, block quality, and injection dynamics.

☑ Current needle placement techniques may need refinement to optimize block efficacy and safety.

☑ Advanced imaging technologies and anatomical understanding are essential to address the limitations of traditional PNB models.

Additional recommended reading

1. McLeod GA, Sadler A, Boezaart A, et al. Peripheral nerve microanatomy: New insights into possible mechanisms for block success. *Reg Anesth Pain Med.* 2024;49:1-14.

2. Reina MA, Boezaart AP, Sala-Blanch X, et al. A novel marker for identifying and studying the membranes, barriers, and compartments surrounding peripheral nerves microscopically. *Clin Anat.* 2018;31:1050-7.

3. Neal JM, Barrington MJ, Brull R, et al. The second ASRA practice advisory on neurologic complications associated with regional anesthesia and pain medicine: Executive summary. *Reg Anesth Pain Med.* 2015;40:401-30.

Fascial plane blocks: From microanatomy to clinical applications

05

Why this topic is important

Fascial plane blocks (FPBs) such as interpectoral plane (IPP) block and pecto-serratus plane (PSP), are a transformative addition to regional anesthesia. They offer effective pain relief with a relatively simple learning curve and a favorable safety profile. They are increasingly utilized across various surgical and nonsurgical settings, from minimally invasive cardiac surgery to chronic pain management.

Understanding the microanatomy of fascia-the connective tissue layers where FPBs are performed-can enhance the clinical application of these blocks (fig-1). This review examines how fascia's cellular and extracellular composition impacts the mechanism of action and effectiveness of FPBs, emphasizing how detailed anatomical knowledge can improve pain management outcomes.

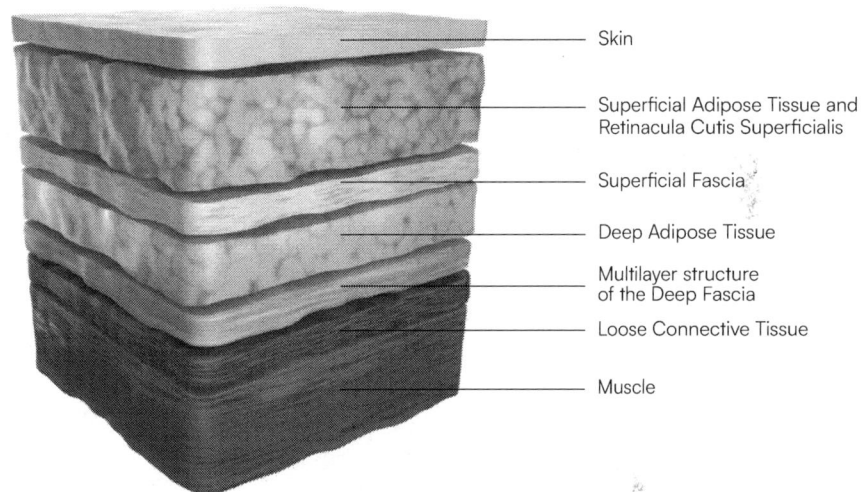

Fig-1. Anatomical cross-section of the layers of soft tissue from skin to muscle, highlighting the key structures: Skin, superficial adipose tissue and retinacula cutis superficialis, superficial fascia, deep adipose tissue, multilayer structure of the deep fascia, loose connective tissue, and muscle layer. Image taken from NYSORA LMS. https://nysoralms.com/

Objectives of this update

- To summarize the microscopic composition of fascia and its relevance to FPBs.

- To explore how fascial microanatomy influences anesthetic spread and block effectiveness.

- To provide practical insights for optimizing FPBs in clinical practice.

What is new

Advances in imaging and molecular biology have revealed that fascia is far more complex than previously understood. It has intricate cellular networks, vascular structures, and biomechanical properties that directly influence the efficacy of FPBs. A recent review by Pirri et al. 2024 links these microscopic findings to clinical outcomes, bridging the gap between anatomy and practice.

Key findings

Microscopic structure of fascia

1. Cellular components:

   - Fascia contains fibroblasts, fasciacytes, and myofibroblasts, which produce extracellular matrix (ECM) components like collagen and hyaluronan (HA).

   - Fasciacytes are specialized cells that regulate the gliding ability of fascial layers by producing HA, a critical component for reducing tissue stiffness and enhancing fluid movement.

2. Extracellular matrix:

   - The ECM is a dynamic network of protein fibers, including type I and III collagen, elastic fibers, and a gelatinous ground substance rich in glycosaminoglycans (GAGs).

   - HA facilitates the diffusion and spread of local anesthetics within the fascial plane, enhancing block effectiveness.

3. Innervation of fascia:

   - Fascia is richly innervated, with free nerve endings and specialized receptors in proprioception, pain perception, and autonomic regulation.

   - These features suggest that fascia itself may serve as a target for analgesia, explaining some of the variability in block outcomes.

Mechanisms of action of FPBs

1. Bulk flow and diffusion:

   - Local anesthetics spread through fascial layers via bulk flow (driven by injection pressure) and diffusion (facilitated by the ECM's permeability).

   - Factors such as fascia thickness, elasticity, and ECM composition influence the extent of anesthetic spread.

2. Vascular absorption:

   - FPBs leverage the vascular and lymphatic networks within the fascia, providing local and systemic analgesic effects.

3. Hydro-dissection:

   - Injection of local anesthetics separates fascial layers, creating potential spaces that enhance the distribution of the anesthetic solution.

Clinical implications

Optimizing FPB performance

- Targeting appropriate fascial layers: Different types of fascia (e.g., aponeurotic versus epimysial) vary in their ability to confine local anesthetics. Understanding these differences can guide block technique.

- Customizing injectate properties: Adjusting local anesthetics' volume, concentration, and temperature can improve spread and reduce densification (viscosity changes in HA).

- Leveraging imaging technologies: Modern ultrasound and other imaging modalities enable precise localization of fascial planes, improving block accuracy and safety.

Practical considerations

- Patient factors: Conditions like obesity, prior surgeries, or fascial remodeling can alter ECM properties and affect block outcomes.

- Surgical applications: FPBs are particularly effective for procedures involving the torso and limbs, offering motor-sparing analgesia that enhances recovery.

Fascial plane blocks: From microanatomy to clinical applications

Limitations and future directions

Study limitations

- Most data are derived from cadaveric or laboratory studies, limiting direct clinical applicability.
- Variability in fascial anatomy among patients poses challenges for standardizing techniques.

Future research

- Investigate the long-term effects of FPBs on chronic pain management.
- Develop targeted interventions to modify fascial properties and improve block outcomes.
- Explore how age-related changes in fascia impact FPB efficacy.

Key takeaways

☑ Fascia's microanatomy, including its cellular and ECM components, plays a critical role in the success of FPBs.

☑ FPBs rely on fascia's unique permeability and gliding properties, which can be optimized by precise injection techniques and tailored anesthetic solutions.

☑ Advances in imaging and molecular biology provide opportunities to enhance the clinical application of FPBs, particularly in challenging cases or complex surgeries.

Additional recommended reading

1. Pirri C, Torre DE, Stecco C. Fascial plane blocks: from microanatomy to clinical applications. *Curr Opin Anesthesiol*. 2024;37(5):526-532.

2. Chin KJ, Lirk P, Hollmann MW, Schwarz SKW. Mechanisms of action of fascial plane blocks: A narrative review. *Reg Anesth Pain Med*. 2021;46:618-628.

3. Stecco C, Stern R, Porzionato A, et al. Hyaluronan within fascia in the etiology of myofascial pain. *Surg Radiol Anat*. 2011;33:891-896.

Risks and prevention strategies for infectious complications following regional anesthesia

06

Why this topic is important

Regional anesthesia (RA) is widely used in various surgical and pain management settings due to its benefits, including effective analgesia, reduced opioid requirements, and improved recovery times. However, RA is not without risks. Infectious complications, although rare, can range from superficial infections to severe central nervous system (CNS) issues like meningitis or epidural abscess.

Understanding these infections' contemporary incidence and risk factors is critical to enhancing patient safety. A recent review by Selvamani et al. 2024 synthesizes the latest data on infectious complications associated with central neuraxial blocks (CNBs) and peripheral nerve blocks (PNBs), offering prevention and risk mitigation insights.

Objectives of this update

- To estimate the incidence of infectious complications associated with CNBs and PNBs.

- To highlight the differences in infection risks between these techniques.

- To discuss strategies to minimize infection risk and improve reporting practices.

What is new

- The recent narrative review by Selvamani et al. 2024 compiles and analyzes data from over 76 studies, presenting pooled incidence rates for infectious complications across various RA techniques. It also explores the disparity in infection rates between CNBs and PNBs and emphasizes the need for standardized reporting to improve prevention efforts.

Key findings

Infection rates by technique

1. Central neuraxial blocks (CNBs):

   - Overall infectious complication rate: 9 per 100,000 blocks.

   - CNS infections (e.g., meningitis, epidural abscess): 2 per 100,000 blocks.

   - Obstetric CNBs show even lower rates: overall infections at 1 per 100,000 and CNS infections at 4 per million.

2. Peripheral nerve blocks (PNBs):

   - Catheter-related infections: 1.8%.

   - Single-injection PNBs had no recorded infections in the limited data available, suggesting lower risk than catheter-based techniques.

Risk factors and mechanisms

1. Patient factors:

   - Diabetes, obesity, and prolonged catheter use (>4 days) are associated with increased risk of infection.

   - Immunosuppression or underlying infections (e.g., urinary tract infections) may also predispose patients to complications.

2. Procedure-related factors:

   - Poor aseptic technique during catheter insertion or maintenance increases infection risk.

   - Tunneling of catheters is associated with fewer infections compared to non-tunneled placement.

3. Site-specific risk:

   - Anatomical locations such as the groin or axilla (common for PNBs) are more prone to contamination than the back (CNBs).

Clinical implications

Reducing infection risks

1. Adherence to aseptic techniques:

   - Strict sterile protocols during insertion and maintenance are paramount.

   - Chlorhexidine-based disinfectants are recommended for skin preparation.

2. Catheter management:

   - Limit catheter duration to ≤4 days when possible.

   - Consider tunneling techniques for epidural and peripheral nerve catheters to reduce contamination risks.

3. Monitoring and follow-up:

   - Daily assessment of catheter insertion sites can help identify early signs of infection.

   - Immediate removal of catheters at the first sign of redness, swelling, or purulent discharge.

Role of prophylaxis

- As suggested by retrospective analyses, single-dose antibiotic prophylaxis may reduce infection rates, especially in prolonged catheter use.

Decision-making for patients

- Practitioners should incorporate infection risk estimates into discussions with patients, especially in populations with higher baseline risk factors, such as diabetics or those undergoing complex surgeries.

Limitations and future directions

Study limitations

- High variability in reporting methods and infection definitions across studies.

- The lack of comprehensive data for single-injection PNBs limits understanding of their infection risks.

Future research

- Develop standardized definitions and reporting systems for infections related to RA.

- Investigate the long-term outcomes of infection prevention strategies, including the role of advanced catheter designs.

- Examine the effectiveness of multimodal infection control practices in diverse clinical settings.

Key takeaways

- ☑ Infectious complications following CNBs are rare, with pooled rates of 9 per 100,000 blocks for overall infections and 2 per 100,000 for CNS infections.

- ☑ PNB catheter infections are more common, emphasizing the need for rigorous aseptic techniques and catheter management.

- ☑ Standardized reporting and evidence-based prevention practices are essential to further reduce infection risks in RA.

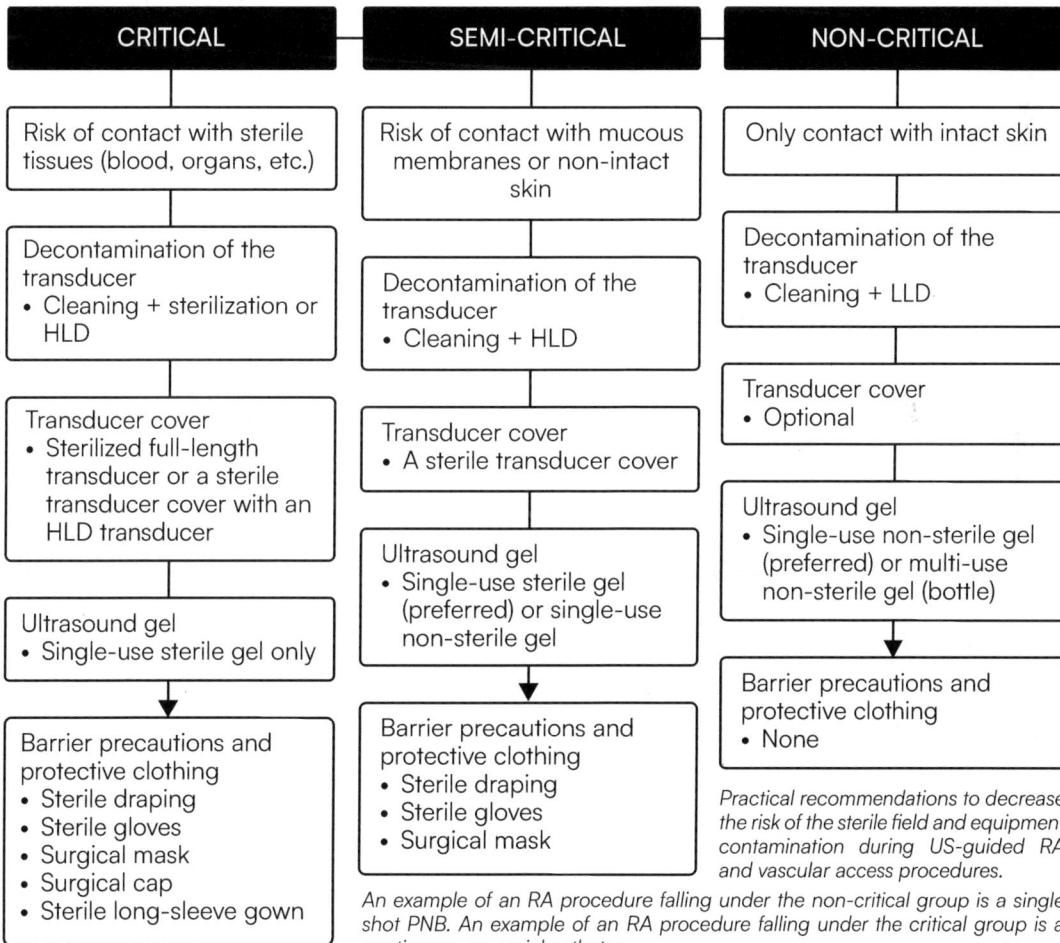

CRITICAL	SEMI-CRITICAL	NON-CRITICAL
Risk of contact with sterile tissues (blood, organs, etc.)	Risk of contact with mucous membranes or non-intact skin	Only contact with intact skin
Decontamination of the transducer • Cleaning + sterilization or HLD	Decontamination of the transducer • Cleaning + HLD	Decontamination of the transducer • Cleaning + LLD
Transducer cover • Sterilized full-length transducer or a sterile transducer cover with an HLD transducer	Transducer cover • A sterile transducer cover	Transducer cover • Optional
Ultrasound gel • Single-use sterile gel only	Ultrasound gel • Single-use sterile gel (preferred) or single-use non-sterile gel	Ultrasound gel • Single-use non-sterile gel (preferred) or multi-use non-sterile gel (bottle)
Barrier precautions and protective clothing • Sterile draping • Sterile gloves • Surgical mask • Surgical cap • Sterile long-sleeve gown	Barrier precautions and protective clothing • Sterile draping • Sterile gloves • Surgical mask	Barrier precautions and protective clothing • None

Practical recommendations to decrease the risk of the sterile field and equipment contamination during US-guided RA and vascular access procedures.

An example of an RA procedure falling under the non-critical group is a single shot PNB. An example of an RA procedure falling under the critical group is a continuous neuraxial catheter.

Additional recommended reading

1. Selvamani BJ, Kalagara H, Volk T, et al. Infectious complications following regional anesthesia: A narrative review and contemporary estimates of risk. *Reg Anesth Pain Med*. 2024;49:1-10.

2. Bomberg H, Bayer I, Wagenpfeil S, et al. Prolonged catheter use and infection in regional anesthesia: A retrospective registry analysis. *Anesthesiology*. 2018;128:764-773.

3. Rosero EB, Joshi GP. Nationwide incidence of serious complications of epidural analgesia in the United States. *Acta Anaesthesiol Scand*. 2016;60:810-820.

4. Eyssen, A., Cops, J., & Hadzic, A. (2023). Review of Strategies to Prevent Infections Related to Ultrasound-Guided Nerve Blocks and Vascular Access. ActA AnAesth. Bel.

Nerve blocks for upper extremities

Intravenous or perineural dexamethasone for analgesia in interscalene brachial plexus blocks

07

Why this topic is important

Interscalene brachial plexus block (IBPB) is a widely utilized regional anesthesia technique for shoulder surgeries to provide prolonged postoperative analgesia (fig-1). It is often combined with adjuvants, such as dexamethasone, to extend the duration of pain relief, minimizing the need for opioids and reducing their associated side effects, such as nausea, vomiting, and respiratory depression.

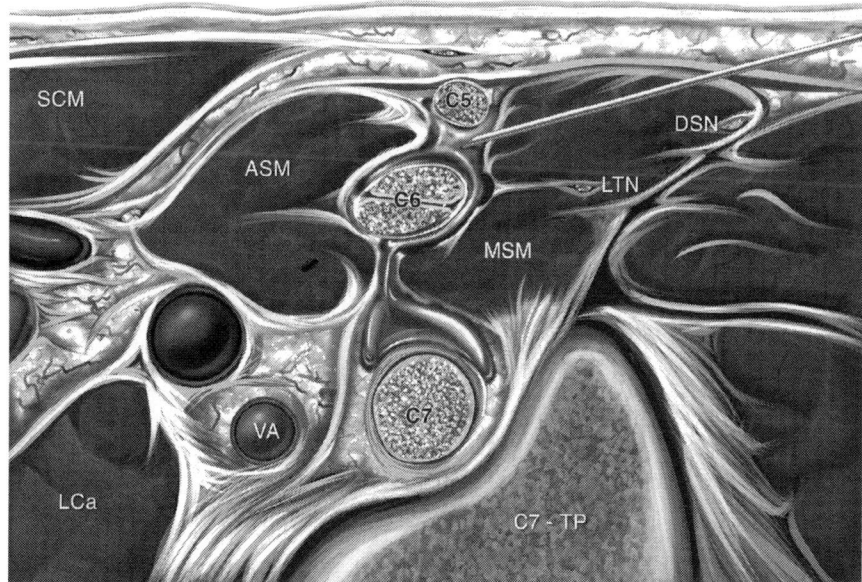

Fig-1. Interscalene block; Reverse ultrasound anatomy with needle insertion in-plane. SCM, sternocleidomastoid; ASM, anterior scalene muscle; LCa, longus capitis muscle; VA, vertebral artery; MSM, middle scalene muscle; LTN, long thoracic nerve; DSN, dorsal scapular nerve; C7-TP, transverse process of C7. Image taken from NYSORA LMS. https://nysoralms.com/

However, there is still uncertainty regarding the optimal route for administering dexamethasone to achieve the most effective and safe outcome. The two primary routes are perineural (injecting the drug near the nerve) and intravenous (IV). Some studies suggest that perineural dexamethasone may provide a longer duration of analgesia compared to IV, but concerns have been raised about the safety and practicality of perineural use. Moreover, the potential risks associated with off-label use and the possibility of drug crystallization when combined with certain local anesthetics like ropivacaine complicate the decision-making process. Given these debates, providing clinicians with updated evidence to guide optimal clinical practice is critical.

Objectives of this update

- Evaluate the effectiveness of perineural versus intravenous dexamethasone in prolonging analgesia after IBPB.

- Discuss the safety concerns associated with perineural dexamethasone, including drug crystallization and off-label use.

- Review recent evidence and provide recommendations for the optimal route of dexamethasone administration in clinical practice.

What is new

A systematic review, meta-analysis, and trial sequential analysis involving 11 trials and 1,145 patients was recently conducted to compare the efficacy of perineural and intravenous dexamethasone when used as adjuncts in IBPB[1]. The analysis primarily focused on the duration of analgesia, and secondary outcomes such as onset of sensory and motor blocks, pain scores, opioid consumption and side effects.

The review concluded that perineural dexamethasone increases the duration of analgesia by an average of 2 hours compared to intravenous dexamethasone. However, this difference in time may not outweigh the possible safety risks of perineural injection. The analysis also found no clinically significant differences in secondary outcomes like cumulative opioid consumption or pain scores beyond 12 hours. With these findings, the authors recommend the use of intravenous dexamethasone due to its comparable efficacy and safer profile.

Main findings

1. Analgesic duration

   ○ Perineural vs intravenous: The meta-analysis found that the duration of analgesia was extended by an average of 2 hours when dexamethasone was administered perineurally rather than intravenously.

   ○ Clinical significance: While a 2-hour extension in analgesia could be advantageous for certain patients, particularly those undergoing longer or more painful surgeries, the marginal benefit might not justify the increased risks. Clinicians must balance the need for extended pain relief with the safety concerns associated with off-label perineural use.

2. Onset of sensory and motor block

   ○ Perineural dexamethasone marginally reduced the time to the onset of both sensory and motor block compared to intravenous administration. However, the difference was small and had no significant clinical impact. Most studies reported only a few minutes of difference, which is unlikely to affect surgical outcomes or overall patient experience meaningfully.

3. Pain scores

   ○ At 12 hours postoperatively, patients receiving perineural dexamethasone reported lower pain scores at rest. However, the two groups had no significant differences in pain scores at 24 or 48 hours. This suggests that the early pain relief advantage of perineural dexamethasone diminishes over time.

4. Opioid consumption

   ○ The cumulative opioid consumption at 24 and 48 hours postoperatively did not differ significantly between the perineural and intravenous dexamethasone groups. This suggests that the slight prolongation of analgesia with perineural dexamethasone does not translate into a meaningful reduction in opioid use, which is one of the primary goals of prolonging regional block analgesia.

5. Glycemic control

   ○ Dexamethasone, whether given intravenously or perineurally, can lead to transient increases in blood glucose levels. However, the differences between the two routes of administration in terms of glycemic impact were minimal, and no significant hyperglycemia-related complications were reported.

Safety concerns

- Crystallization risk: One of the major concerns with perineural dexamethasone is the risk of drug crystallization when combined with certain local anesthetics, such as ropivacaine. Crystallization can cause nerve damage, resulting in serious complications like persistent paraesthesia or even nerve injury. Although crystallization can be avoided by administering the drugs sequentially rather than mixed, the potential for in situ crystallization remains a risk.

- Off-label use: Perineural administration of dexamethasone is considered off-label, meaning regulatory bodies have not formally approved it for this specific use. Although studies to date have shown no major safety concerns, the off-label status introduces legal and ethical considerations that clinicians must weigh when deciding the route of administration.

Challenges and limitations

1. Low quality of evidence:

   - Many trials had small sample sizes and limited power, leading to low-confidence ratings for some outcomes.

2. Generalizability:

   - Findings were specific to IBPB, and results may not apply to other nerve blocks.

3. Lack of long-term data:

   - No data on chronic pain outcomes or late-onset complications were reported.

Key takeaways

☑ Perineural dexamethasone extends analgesia by about two hours compared to intravenous dexamethasone, but the clinical significance of this is limited.

☑ Perineural administration is associated with risks such as drug crystallization and is considered off-label, making intravenous dexamethasone the safer and more practical option in most cases.

☑ There are no significant differences in opioid consumption, pain on movement, or overall patient satisfaction between the two routes.

☑ Intravenous dexamethasone offers nearly equivalent pain relief while avoiding the potential complications of perineural injection, making it the recommended route for most patients undergoing IBPB.

☑ For patients requiring extended analgesia, alternatives to dexamethasone or other multimodal analgesia strategies should be considered to enhance safety and effectiveness.

Additional recommended reading

1. Albrecht E, Renard Y, Desai N. Intravenous versus perineural dexamethasone to prolong analgesia after interscalene brachial plexus block: A systematic review with meta-analysis and trial sequential analysis. *Br J Anaesth*. 2024;133(1):135-145.

2. Desai N, Kirkham KR, Albrecht E. Local anaesthetic adjuncts for peripheral regional anaesthesia: *A narrative review. Anaesthesia.* 2021;76(Suppl 1):100-109.

3. Hussain N, Brummett CM, et al. Equivalent analgesic effectiveness between perineural and intravenous dexamethasone as adjuvants for peripheral nerve blockade: A systematic review and meta-analysis. *Can J Anaesth*. 2018;65(2):194-206.

Mixture of bupivacaine-lidocaine or bupivacaine alone for infraclavicular block

08

Why this topic is important

Ultrasound-guided infraclavicular brachial plexus blocks (ICBPBs) are widely used for upper- extremities surgeries, providing effective intraoperative anesthesia and postoperative analgesia (fig-1). While effective, one of the challenges clinicians face with peripheral nerve blocks is the balance between rapid onset and prolonged analgesia. Local anesthetics like bupivacaine are favored for their long-lasting effects, but they can have a delayed onset, potentially affecting surgical efficiency. In contrast, adding faster-acting agents like lidocaine to long-acting anesthetics can accelerate onset, though this often shortens the duration of the block.

Understanding the implications of anesthetic choice-whether to use a long-acting local anesthetic alone or combine it with a faster-acting one-can improve patient outcomes, optimize pain management, and potentially reduce the need for additional analgesics postoperatively. Therefore, comparing the efficacy and characteristics of a mixture of bupivacaine and lidocaine versus bupivacaine alone in infraclavicular blocks offers valuable insights for improving anesthetic care during upper extremity surgeries.

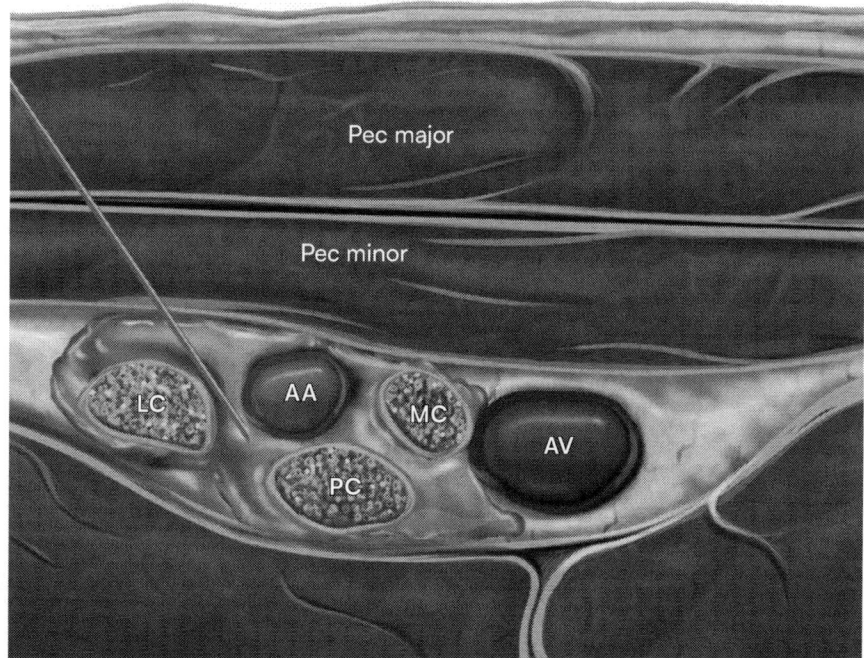

Fig-1. Infraclavicular brachial plexus block, reverse ultrasound anatomy with needle insertion in-plane. Local anesthetic spread around the axillary artery. AA, axillary artery; AV, axillary vein; LC, lateral cord; MC, medial cord; PC, posterior cord.
Image taken from NYSORA LMS. https://nysoralms.com/

Objectives of this update

- To compare the clinical outcomes of using 0.25% bupivacaine combined with 1% lidocaine against 0.5% bupivacaine alone in ICBPBs.

- To assess how the combination of local anesthetics affects the duration of motor and sensory block, as well as the duration of postoperative analgesia.

- To examine the trade-offs between block onset time and overall duration of analgesia to inform clinical decision-making.

- To provide recommendations for anesthetic strategies based on the surgical context and patient needs.

What is new

A recent randomized controlled trial by Aguilera et al. (2024)[1] aimed to assess the differences between a mixture of 0.25% bupivacaine with 1% lidocaine versus 0.5% bupivacaine for ultrasound-guided infraclavicular brachial plexus blocks. A total of 40 patients scheduled for upper extremity surgery were randomized into two groups: one group receiving the bupivacaine-lidocaine mixture and the other receiving bupivacaine alone. Both groups also received perineural adjuvants (epinephrine and dexamethasone) to prolong the block's effect.

The key findings of the study are as follows:

- Prolonged block duration with bupivacaine alone: Compared to the mixed solution, 0.5% bupivacaine significantly extended the duration of both motor and sensory blocks. Motor block duration was prolonged by approximately 9.5 hours, and sensory block duration was 10.6 hours, offering patients longer periods of postoperative pain relief.

- Faster onset with bupivacaine-lidocaine mixture: Patients receiving the bupivacaine-lidocaine mixture experienced a faster onset of block (within 20 minutes), whereas those receiving bupivacaine alone had a slower onset time (around 35 minutes).

- Extended postoperative analgesia: The duration of postoperative analgesia was substantially longer in the bupivacaine-only group, lasting on average 14 hours longer than in the mixed group.

- Incidence of rebound pain: Rebound pain, defined as severe pain occurring once the nerve block resolves, was observed less

frequently in the 0.5% bupivacaine group (11.1%) compared to the bupivacaine-lidocaine mixture group (31.6%).

Trial design and methodology

This prospective, randomized, double-blind study recruited 40 patients undergoing distal upper extremity surgeries (e.g., forearm, wrist, or hand fractures) at the Hospital de San Carlos in Chile. The patients were randomly assigned to two groups:

- Group BL: Received a mixture of 0.25% bupivacaine and 1% lidocaine.

- Group B: Received 0.5% bupivacaine.

Both groups received the same total volume of anesthetic (35 mL) along with perineural adjuvants (epinephrine and dexamethasone) to enhance the block's effect. All blocks were performed by the same experienced anesthesiologist using a standardized ultrasound-guided infraclavicular technique.

The primary outcome was motor block duration, while secondary outcomes included sensory block duration, onset time, duration of postoperative analgesia, and incidence of rebound pain.

Results

1. Motor block duration: The mean motor block duration in the 0.5% bupivacaine group was *28.4 hours,* significantly longer than in the bupivacaine-lidocaine mixture group *(18.9 hours).* This represents an extension of 50% in block duration when using bupivacaine alone.

2. Sensory block duration: Similarly, the sensory block lasted *29.3 hours* in the bupivacaine group versus *18.7 hours* in the mixed group, a difference of over 10 hours in favor of the bupivacaine-alone approach.

3. Postoperative analgesia duration: The 0.5% bupivacaine group experienced notably longer postoperative analgesia, lasting 38.3 hours, compared to the 24.3 hours in the mixed group. This extended analgesic

effect greatly benefits patients, reducing the need for supplementary pain medication postoperatively.

4. Onset time: While the bupivacaine-alone strategy resulted in longer block and analgesia duration, the onset time was slower, taking approximately *35 minutes* compared to *20 minutes* in the mixed anesthetic group. This quicker onset with the bupivacaine-lidocaine combination may be useful in settings where a rapid anesthetic effect is required.

5. Rebound pain: Though not statistically significant, there was a trend toward reduced rebound pain in the bupivacaine-alone group (11.1% vs. 31.6%). Rebound pain can be a distressing experience for patients as the block wears off, leading to increased postoperative pain intensity. The study's results suggest that longer-lasting blocks may reduce the incidence of this phenomenon, potentially due to the slower, more gradual resolution of anesthesia.

6. Adverse events: There were no significant differences between the groups regarding adverse effects such as vascular puncture, paresthesia, or local anesthetic systemic toxicity (LAST).

Key outcome measures.

Outcome	Bupivacaine-lidocaine (0.25% - 1%)	Bupivacaine (0.5%)	Difference
Motor block duration (hours)	18.9	28.4	+9.5 hours
Sensory block duration (hours)	18.7	29.3	+10.6 hours
Postoperative analgesia (hours)	24.3	38.3	+14 hours
Onset time (Minutes)	20	35	-15 minutes
Rebound pain incidence	31.6%	11.1%	Lower by 20.5%

Clinical implications and decision-making

- Prolonged surgeries or intense postoperative pain:
  For longer surgeries or cases where significant postoperative pain is anticipated (e.g., bone surgery), 0.5% bupivacaine should be favored due to its prolonged analgesic effect, which reduces the need for postoperative opioids or rescue analgesics.

- When rapid onset is crucial: The bupivacaine-lidocaine mixture may be more suitable in surgical settings where the block needs to be established quickly (e.g., in urgent cases). This combination offers the benefit of faster onset, which can help minimize surgical delays.

- Managing rebound pain: The incidence of rebound pain was lower in the bupivacaine group, highlighting the potential advantages of prolonged blocks in reducing this adverse effect. Clinicians should consider longer-lasting anesthetic techniques, particularly in outpatient settings where patients may experience intense pain as the block wears off.

- Block performance and optimization: The study reaffirms that using 0.5% bupivacaine in combination with adjuvants like dexamethasone and epinephrine can optimize the performance of ICBPBs. This combination yields a strong balance of sensory and motor block duration while minimizing the occurrence of rebound pain and extending postoperative analgesia.

Recommendations for practice

- For surgeries requiring prolonged post-operative analgesia:
  Use 0.5% bupivacaine for patients requiring long-lasting postoperative pain relief. This can be particularly useful in cases where additional postoperative opioid use is to be minimized.

- When time is of the essence: In situations requiring a rapid onset of anesthesia, the bupivacaine-lidocaine mixture may be preferred. This strategy works well in busy operating rooms or emergency cases where time is critical.

- Multimodal analgesia for rebound pain: Given the higher incidence of rebound pain in the bupivacaine-lidocaine group, employing multimodal analgesic techniques (e.g., non-opioid analgesics, gabapentinoids) may mitigate the impact of block resolution and enhance patient comfort postoperatively.

Key takeaways

☑ 0.5% bupivacaine significantly prolongs motor and sensory block duration compared to the bupivacaine-lidocaine mixture.

☑ The bupivacaine-lidocaine mixture provides a faster onset but shorter block and analgesic durations.

☑ Clinicians should balance the need for fast onset and prolonged postoperative pain relief when choosing an anesthetic.

☑ Adjuvants like dexamethasone may help extend the duration of both sensory and motor blocks and reduce the likelihood of rebound pain.

Additional recommended reading

1. Aguilera G, Tabilo C, Jara Á, et al. 0.25% Bupivacaine—1% Lidocaine vs 0.5% Bupivacaine for Ultrasound-Guided Infraclavicular Brachial Plexus Block: A Randomized Controlled Trial. *Reg Anesth Pain Med.* 2024;0:1-8.

2. Aliste J, Layera S, Bravo D, et al. Randomized comparison between perineural dexamethasone and dexmedetomidine for ultrasound-guided infraclavicular block. *Reg Anesth Pain Med.* 2019;44:911-6.

3. Veena G, Pangotra A, Kumar S, et al. Comparison of perineural and intravenous dexamethasone as an adjuvant to levobupivacaine in ultrasound-guided infraclavicular brachial plexus block. *Anesth Essays Res.* 2021;15:45-50.

Anterior glenoid block as an alternative to interscalene brachial plexus block

09

Why this topic is important

Shoulder surgeries, such as arthroscopic rotator cuff repair, frequently necessitate regional anesthesia to provide effective perioperative analgesia. The interscalene brachial plexus block (ISB) is the gold standard for these procedures due to its excellent analgesia. However, ISB is associated with a significant risk of phrenic nerve palsy, leading to diaphragmatic paralysis, which limits its application in patients with compromised respiratory function.

Emerging alternatives, such as the anterior glenoid block (AGB), aim to provide comparable analgesia while minimizing complications. The AGB targets articular branches of the axillary and subscapular nerves, which supply the glenohumeral joint, and avoids the proximal brachial plexus, thus preserving diaphragmatic function. This makes AGB particularly valuable for high-risk patients or those in outpatient settings where motor-sparing and early recovery are prioritized.

This update explores the AGB as an innovative approach for shoulder surgery analgesia, emphasizing its potential benefits, practical considerations, and areas for further investigation.

Objectives of this update

- Describe the anterior glenoid block and its anatomical targets.

- Compare its clinical outcomes with interscalene brachial plexus block.

- Discuss its applicability in diverse patient populations and clinical scenarios.

What is new

A recent study[1] evaluated the AGB combined with a selective anterior suprascapular nerve block in 45 patients undergoing arthroscopic rotator cuff repair. Key findings include:

- Effective analgesia, with 87% of patients reporting mild pain (NRS ≤ 4) within 24 hours postoperatively.

- Preservation of diaphragmatic function and handgrip strength in most patients.

- No reported complications, such as nerve damage, infection, or hematoma.

Detailed findings

Anatomy and technique

The AGB targets the articular branches of the axillary and subscapular nerves, located deep to the subscapularis muscle at the anterior glenoid margin. This approach avoids the phrenic nerve and brachial plexus trunks, minimizing motor and diaphragmatic impairment.

Procedure:

- The patient is placed supine, and a curvilinear transducer is positioned parallel to the clavicle.

- Under ultrasound guidance, the needle is advanced medially through the deltoid and subscapularis muscles to the anterior glenoid.

- Local anesthetic (15 mL of ropivacaine 0.5%) is injected at the articular margin, ensuring diffusion beneath the subscapularis.

The AGB is frequently paired with an anterior suprascapular nerve block for enhanced analgesia, targeting the acromioclavicular joint.

Clinical outcomes

1. Pain scores:

   ◦ Median NRS pain scores were consistently mild (≤ 4) at 4, 8, and 24 hours postoperatively.

2. Preserved function:

   ◦ Diaphragmatic function: 87% of patients retained > 80% of their baseline diaphragmatic excursion amplitude under ultrasonography.

   ◦ Handgrip strength:
   Similarly, 87% maintained > 80% of baseline handgrip strength, underscoring the motor-sparing nature of the block.

3. Safety:

   ◦ No adverse events, including bleeding, hematoma, infection, or nerve damage, were observed in the study cohort.

Implications for practice

Advantages of the anterior glenoid block

- Phrenic nerve sparing: Unlike ISB, the AGB does not compromise diaphragmatic function, making it suitable for patients with respiratory limitations.

- Motor-sparing: Preserved handgrip strength allows for early mobilization and functional recovery.

- Reduced complication risk: Avoidance of proximal plexus structures minimizes the risk of pneumothorax, Horner's syndrome, and other ISB-associated complications.

Patient selection

1. Ideal candidates:

   ◦ Patients with chronic obstructive pulmonary disease (COPD), obesity, or other conditions where phrenic nerve paralysis poses significant risk.

   ◦ Outpatient surgery patients who benefit from faster recovery and functional preservation.

2. Limitations:

   ◦ The AGB does not address lateral shoulder pain effectively, which may limit its standalone use in broader surgical contexts.

Procedural considerations

- Ultrasound Expertise:
  Successful implementation requires advanced ultrasound skills to identify the anterior glenoid and ensure accurate needle placement.

- Adjunct Techniques: Pairing with anterior suprascapular nerve block enhances coverage for the acromioclavicular joint, extending its utility.

Challenges and limitations

1. Limited evidence base:

   ◦ While promising, current data on the AGB are derived from single-center studies with modest sample sizes. Larger, randomized trials are needed to establish efficacy and safety profiles.

2. Learning curve:

   ◦ Mastering the AGB requires familiarity with shoulder anatomy and ultrasound techniques, which may limit adoption in resource-limited settings.

3. Comparison with other techniques:

   ◦ Direct comparisons with other regional blocks, such as the ISB, costoclavicular block, or posterior suprascapular nerve block, are necessary to delineate relative advantages.

Key takeaways

☑ The anterior glenoid block is a promising alternative to interscalene brachial plexus block, offering effective analgesia with reduced risk of phrenic nerve palsy.

☑ It preserves diaphragmatic function and motor strength, making it ideal for high-risk or outpatient populations.

☑ Combining AGB with the anterior suprascapular nerve block enhances its coverage and utility.

Additional recommended reading

1. Xu C, Wang C, Xu Y, et al. Anterior glenoid block as an alternative technique to interscalene brachial plexus block. *Anesth Analg.* 2024;138(2):483-484.

2. El-Boghdadly K, Chin KJ, Chan VWS. Phrenic nerve palsy and regional anesthesia for shoulder surgery: anatomical, physiologic, and clinical considerations. *Anesthesiology.* 2017;127(2):173-191.

3. Tran J, Peng PWH, Agur AMR. Anatomical study of the innervation of glenohumeral and acromioclavicular joint capsules: implications for image-guided intervention. *Reg Anesth Pain Med.* 2019;44:237-244..

Local anesthetic spread in clavipectoral fascia plane block

10

Why this topic is important

Fractures of the clavicle often necessitate effective anesthesia techniques to manage pain and facilitate surgical intervention. While interscalene brachial plexus block (IBPB) is the traditional choice, its associated risks, such as phrenic nerve palsy, pose challenges, particularly for patients with respiratory compromise. The clavipectoral fascia plane block (CPB) offers an alternative approach, targeting clavicular innervation while avoiding complications linked to deeper nerve blocks (fig-1). A recent study by Labandeyra et al. examines the anatomical spread of CPB, providing critical insights into its potential efficacy for clavicle-related surgeries and its ability to provide focused analgesia without affecting deeper structures.

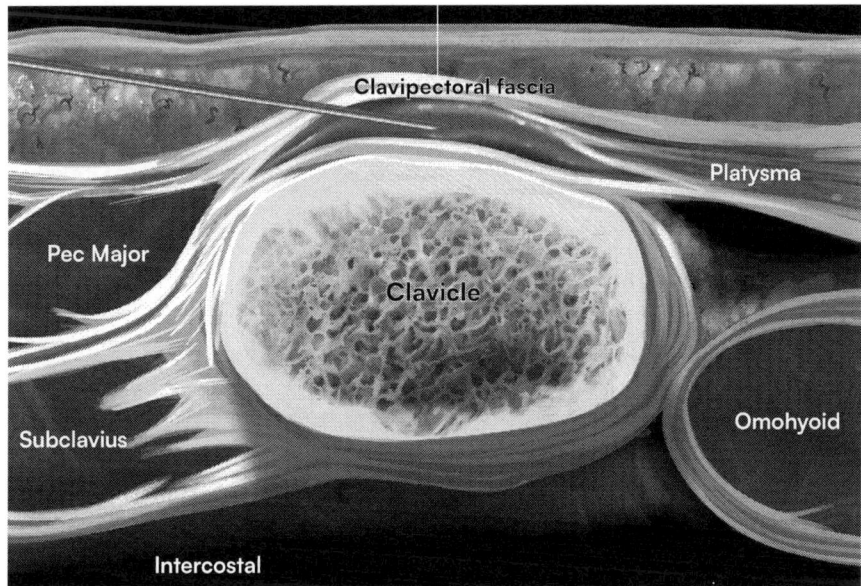

Fig-1. Clavipectoral fascia plane block, reverse ultrasound anatomy with needle insertion in-plane. Image taken from NYSORA LMS. https://nysoralms.com/

Objectives of this update

- To investigate the distribution of local anesthetic solution using CPB in cadaveric models.

- To determine its effectiveness in targeting the clavicular periosteum and superficial muscular planes.

- To identify potential limitations in its anatomical coverage.

What is new

The study by Labandeyra et al. is the first detailed anatomical study to clarify the distribution patterns of CPB. The findings indicate effective staining of the anterosuperior clavicular periosteum and supraclavicular nerves while sparing deeper muscular planes, including the clavipectoral fascia (CPF).

Study findings

Methodology

- Design: Cadaveric anatomical study using 12 clavicle samples from 6 cadavers.

- Intervention: CPB was performed using ultrasound guidance, injecting 20 mL of a methylene blue and iodinated contrast solution at two points along the clavicle.

- Assessment: Dissections and CT scans evaluated the distribution of the injected solution across superficial and deep anatomical planes.

Key results

1. Superficial and periosteal staining

   - The injected solution consistently stained the medial, intermediate, and lateral supraclavicular nerves (90%).

   - Staining was observed in the superficial muscular plane, including the deltoid (100%), trapezius (100%), sternocleidomastoid (60%), and pectoralis major muscles (100%).

   - The anterosuperior periosteum of the clavicle was stained in 53.5% of its surface, while the posteroinferior periosteum showed minimal staining (4%).

2. Deep muscular plane and CPF

   - No staining was observed in deeper structures such as the subclavius muscle, pectoralis minor, or CPF.

- These findings suggest that CPB does not effectively reach deeper clavicular regions or the CPF, contrary to earlier assumptions about its anatomical coverage.

3. Imaging correlation

   - CT scans confirmed consistent staining in the anterosuperior periclavicular region, aligning with observations from anatomical dissections.

   - Both imaging and dissection demonstrated limited solution spread beyond superficial planes, reinforcing CPB's focused action.

Clinical implications

Advantages of CPB

- CPB effectively targets supraclavicular nerves and superficial clavicular structures, providing focused analgesia for clavicle surgeries.

- Its avoidance of deeper structures reduces the risk of complications associated with IBPB, such as phrenic nerve palsy.

Limitations of CPB

- Limited staining of deeper structures, such as the CPF and posteroinferior clavicular periosteum, suggests it may not provide comprehensive analgesia for all clavicular fractures.

- CPB may be less effective for surgeries requiring extensive periosteal coverage or deep tissue analgesia.

Practical considerations

- CPB is a straightforward block with clearly defined ultrasound landmarks and minimal associated risks.

- Ideal for patients who require clavicle surgery but are at high risk of respiratory complications from IBPB.

Limitations and future directions

Study limitations

- Cadaveric nature: Findings may only partially translate to in vivo conditions due to differences in tissue elasticity and vascular dynamics.

- Small sample size: A limited number of cadavers restricts the generalizability of results.

- Unfractured clavicles: Results may differ in fractured or surgically altered anatomy.

Recommendations for future research

- Clinical trials are needed to evaluate the analgesic effectiveness of CPB in live patients undergoing clavicle surgery.

- Studies assessing modifications to the CPB technique to enhance deep plane coverage could expand its clinical utility.

Key takeaways

- ☑ CPB effectively distributes anesthetic solution to the anterosuperior clavicular periosteum, superficial muscles, and supraclavicular nerves.

- ☑ Deeper structures, including the CPF and posteroinferior periosteum, remain unstained, limiting its coverage for some clavicular surgeries.

- ☑ CPB provides a safer alternative to IBPB, particularly for patients at risk of respiratory complications, but may require adjunctive techniques for broader analgesic coverage.

Additional recommended reading

1. Labandeyra H, Heredia-Carques C, Campoy JC, et al. Clavipectoral fascia plane block spread: An anatomical study. *Reg Anesth Pain Med.* 2024;49(4):368-372.

2. Valdés-Vilches L, et al. Ultrasound-guided clavipectoral fascia plane block: A case series. *Rev Esp Anestesiol Reanim.* 2022;69:683-8.

3. Zhuo Q, Zheng Y, Hu Z, et al. Ultrasound-guided clavipectoral fascia block for clavicular surgery: A randomized controlled trial. *Anesth Analg.* 2022;135:633-40.

Interscalene block with and without superficial cervical plexus block in clavicle surgery

11

Why this topic is important

Clavicle fractures are a common orthopedic injury, with some cases requiring surgical intervention. Regional anesthesia (RA) offers a safer alternative to general anesthesia (GA), avoiding complications like nausea, vomiting, and hemodynamic stress. Interscalene block (ISB) is widely used for clavicle surgery, often combined with superficial cervical plexus block (SCPB) to enhance coverage of the clavicle's complex innervation (fig-1). However, the necessity of SCPB alongside ISB remains to be determined. A recent study by Mosaffa et al. evaluates whether ISB alone is as effective as ISB combined with SCPB in providing adequate anesthesia and analgesia for clavicle surgery.

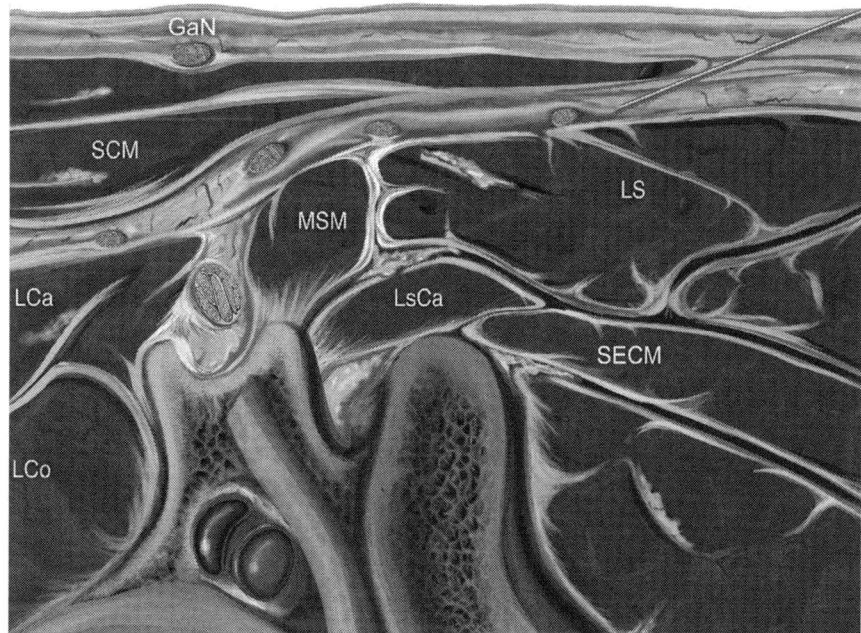

Fig-1. Cervical plexus block; Reverse ultrasound anatomy. GaN, greater auricular nerve; SCM, sternocleidomastoid muscle; LCa, longus capitis muscle; LCo, longus Colli muscle; MSM, middle scalene muscle; LsCa, longissimus capitis muscle; LS, levator scapulae muscle; SECM, semispinalis capitis muscle. *Image taken from NYSORA LMS. https://nysoralms.com/*

Objectives of this update

- To compare the efficacy of ISB with and without SCPB in providing adequate anesthesia for clavicle surgery.

- To assess outcomes, including pain scores, sedation requirements, opioid consumption, and conversion to general anesthesia.

- To determine if SCPB enhances analgesia or reduces postoperative discomfort compared to ISB alone.

What is new

This randomized, double-blind clinical trial by Mofassa et al. 2024 demonstrates that ISB alone is equally effective as ISB combined with SCPB in providing anesthesia and analgesia for clavicle fracture surgery. The findings suggest that SCPB may not be necessary for most patients undergoing this procedure.

Key findings

Study design and population

Participants: 120 patients undergoing clavicle surgery randomized into two groups: ISB alone or ISB + SCPB.

- Methodology:

  ◦ ISB performed under ultrasound guidance with 20 mL of 1.5% lidocaine, bicarbonate, epinephrine, and 0.5% bupivacaine.

  ◦ SCPB used an additional 10 mL of the same anesthetic mixture.

- Primary outcome: Conversion to GA.

- Secondary outcomes: Pain scores (VAS), sedation requirements, and opioid consumption in the PACU.

Results

1. Conversion to GA

   ◦ No patients in either group required conversion to GA, confirming the adequacy of both approaches for clavicle surgery.

2. Pain scores (VAS)

   ◦ There was no significant difference in mean VAS scores in PACU, suggesting comparable analgesic efficacy.

3. Sedation requirements

   ◦ Rates of additional sedation (midazolam 2 mg or fentanyl 50 μg) were similar in both groups.

4. Opioid consumption

   ◦ Meperidine usage in the PACU was identical in both groups.

5. Other findings

   ◦ There were no significant differences between the groups in surgery duration, nerve block initiation time, or surgery initiation time.

   ◦ No adverse events were reported in either group.

Clinical implications

Simplifying regional anesthesia for clavicle surgery

The results demonstrate that ISB alone is sufficient for most clavicle surgeries, challenging the necessity of routinely adding SCPB. This simplifies the anesthetic approach, reducing procedure time and the complexity of the block technique.

Advantages of ISB alone

- Streamlined block procedure: Without the additional SCPB, block administration is faster, and practitioners can focus solely on achieving a high-quality ISB.

- Safety profile: SCPB carries a small risk of phrenic nerve involvement or complications such as neck hematoma. Avoiding SCPB reduces these risks.

- Resource efficiency: Eliminating SCPB conserves anesthetic volume and reduces total drug exposure.

Situations where SCPB may still be beneficial

While this study suggests that SCPB is unnecessary for most cases, there may be instances where SCPB could be valuable:

- Complex clavicle fractures involving extensive soft tissue damage or requiring longer surgical durations.

- Patients with incomplete analgesia from ISB alone, although such cases were not observed in this study.

Practical recommendations

1. Routine practice: ISB alone should be considered the first-line regional technique for clavicle surgeries, offering effective anesthesia and analgesia with a simpler protocol.

2. Individualized approach: SCPB can be added selectively if the initial ISB fails to provide adequate coverage or the surgical team anticipates extended operative times.

3. Ultrasound guidance: Ultrasound ensures precise block placement, improving efficacy and reducing complications.

Limitations

- Patient selection: The study focused on healthy adults; results may differ in elderly or high-risk patients.

- Short follow-up period: Outcomes were assessed primarily during PACU stay, with no long-term pain or recovery data.

- Limited surgical variability: The findings may not apply to more complex clavicle surgeries requiring extensive soft tissue manipulation.

Key takeaways

☑ ISB alone provides anesthesia equivalent to ISB combined with SCPB for clavicle surgery.

☑ No differences were observed in pain scores, sedation requirements, or opioid consumption between the groups.

☑ Eliminating SCPB simplifies the anesthetic approach, reducing procedure time and risks without compromising efficacy.

☑ SCPB may still have a role in select cases involving complex fractures or inadequate coverage with ISB alone.

Additional recommended reading

1. Mosaffa F, Ghasemi M, Habibi A, et al. Efficacy comparison between interscalene block with and without superficial cervical plexus block for anesthesia in clavicle surgery. *Anesth Pain Med.* 2024;14(1):e142051.

2. Abdelghany MS, Ahmed SA, Afandy ME. Superficial cervical plexus block alone or combined with interscalene brachial plexus block in surgery for clavicle fractures: A randomized clinical trial. *Minerva Anestesiol.* 2021;87(5):523-32.

3. Gupta N, Gupta V, Kumar G, et al. Comparative evaluation of interscalene block vs. interscalene block and superficial cervical plexus block for clavicular fractures. *Int J Contemp Med Res.* 2019;6(3):822-30.

Regional anesthesia for lower extremities

PENG block or suprainguinal fascia iliaca block for hip fracture pain

12

Why this topic is important

Hip fractures are common in elderly populations and are often associated with significant dynamic pain, especially during movement or positioning. This pain can impair the patient's ability to achieve appropriate positions for spinal anesthesia, delay surgical interventions, and negatively affect overall outcomes. Effective preoperative pain control reduces stress responses, stabilizes hemodynamics, and improves patient comfort.

Peripheral nerve blocks are pivotal in multimodal analgesia for hip fractures. They provide superior pain relief, decrease opioid consumption, and reduce opioid-related side effects such as respiratory depression and delirium, which are particularly concerning in older patients. Among these techniques, the suprainguinal fascia iliaca compartment block (SIFICB) is widely used for its efficacy in alleviating dynamic pain by targeting the femoral nerve and lateral femoral cutaneous nerve (LFCN) (fig-1A).

A newer approach, the pericapsular nerve group (PENG) block, specifically targets articular branches of the femoral, obturator, and accessory obturator nerves innervating the anterior hip capsule (fig-1B). Its motor-sparing properties make it an attractive option for hip fracture management. However, limited data directly compare its efficacy with established blocks like SIFICB, particularly for dynamic pain.

A recent study by Koh et al.[1] evaluates the relative effectiveness of the PENG block and SIFICB in managing dynamic pain and explores their implications for clinical practice.

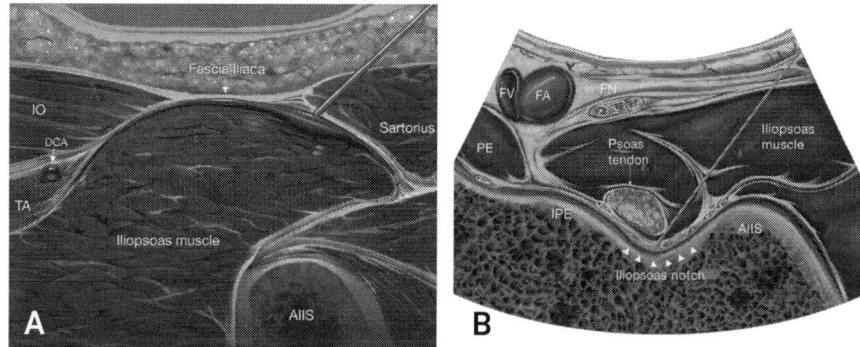

Fig-1A. Reverse ultrasound anatomy for a suprainguinal approach to a fascia iliaca block. Needle insertion is shown in-plane with LA distribution (blue) under the fascia iliaca. AIIS, anterior inferior iliac spine; IO, internal oblique; TA, transversus abdominis; DCA, deep circumflex artery. Fig-1B. Pericapsular nerve group (PENG) block, reverse ultrasound anatomy. Local anesthetic spread in the plane between the iliopsoas muscle and pubic ramus and the anterior capsule of the hip, thereby anesthetizing the articular branches of the femoral, obturator, and accessory obturator nerves. FA, femoral artery; FV, femoral vein; FN, femoral nerve; PE, pectineus muscle; IPE, iliopubic eminence; AIIS, anterior inferior iliac spine. Image taken from NYSORA LMS. https://nysoralms.com/

Objectives of this update

- Compare the effectiveness of the PENG block and SIFICB in reducing dynamic pain in hip fracture patients.

- Assess additional outcomes, including postoperative pain, motor function, recovery profiles, and complications.

- Highlight practical considerations for selecting nerve blocks in hip fracture management.

What is new

The randomized controlled trial by Koh et al.[1] is among the first to directly compare the analgesic effects of the PENG block and SIFICB in hip fracture patients. Key features include:

- Evaluation of dynamic pain reduction 30 minutes after block administration.

- Secondary outcomes include postoperative pain scores, motor function, recovery milestones, and complications.

- Use standardized block volumes (20 mL ropivacaine 0.3% for PENG; 30 mL ropivacaine 0.3% for SIFICB).

Detailed findings

Study design

This single-center study enrolled 80 adult patients undergoing hip fracture surgery. All participants reported baseline dynamic pain scores ≥ 4 on a numerical rating scale (NRS). They were randomized into two groups: PENG block (n=40) or SIFICB (n=40). Dynamic pain scores were measured during passive leg raising.

Primary outcome: Dynamic pain reduction

Both the PENG block and SIFICB significantly reduced dynamic pain, but there was no significant difference between the two groups:

- Pain reduction after PENG block: 3.1 NRS points.

- Pain reduction after SIFICB: 2.9 NRS points.

Secondary outcomes

1. Dynamic and resting pain:

   ○ Both blocks provided comparable pain relief at 6, 24, and 48 hours postoperatively.

2. Motor function:

   ○ Post-block motor function was preserved in both groups, with no significant differences in Bromage scores or ambulation tests.

3. Recovery profiles:

   ○ The groups ' time to ambulation, urinary catheter removal, and hospital discharge were similar.

4. Complications:

   ○ There are no significant differences in postoperative complications, including cognitive dysfunction, delirium, or acute kidney injury.

Implications for practice

Block efficacy and safety

The PENG block and SIFICB effectively manage dynamic pain in hip fracture patients. Their comparable efficacy suggests that either can be incorporated into preoperative pain management protocols.

Patient selection and block choice

Consider PENG block when:

- Motor-sparing is a priority, such as in patients at high risk of falls.

- Localized anterior hip capsule pain is predominant.

Consider SIFICB when:

- Broad coverage of the LFCN is required, such as for lateral thigh pain associated with certain surgical incisions.

Practical considerations

- The volume of anesthetic: Adequate injectate volume is critical for fascial plane blocks like SIFICB to ensure effective coverage of the lumbar plexus.
- Block timing: Both blocks demonstrated analgesic effects within 30 minutes, making them suitable for preoperative use in routine clinical workflows.

Challenges and limitations

Lack of long-term data:

- This study focused on early postoperative outcomes. Further research is needed to explore long-term effects on functional recovery and chronic pain.

Cognitive function in elderly patients:

- Older patients may struggle to report pain scores accurately, potentially influencing the study's findings. However, complementary verbal scales and objective measures addressed this limitation.

Anatomical variability:

- Injectate spread and effectiveness can vary based on individual anatomy, particularly for fascial plane blocks.

Key takeaways

☑ The PENG block and SIFICB are equally effective in reducing dynamic pain in hip fracture patients.

☑ Both blocks preserve motor function, making them safe options for elderly patients.

☑ Patient-specific factors, including pain location and surgical approach should guide block choice.

☑ Early implementation of nerve blocks can enhance patient comfort and streamline preoperative care.

Additional recommended reading

1. Koh WU, Kim H, Kim YJ, et al. Comparison of analgesic effect of pericapsular nerve group block and suprainguinal fascia iliaca compartment block on dynamic pain in patients with hip fractures: A randomized controlled trial. *Reg Anesth Pain Med.* 2024;0:1-6.

2. Girón-Arango L, Peng PWH, Chin KJ, et al. Pericapsular nerve group (PENG) block for hip fracture. *Reg Anesth Pain Med.* 2018;43:859-63.

3. Vermeylen K, Desmet M, Leunen I, et al. Suprainguinal injection for fascia iliaca compartment block results in more consistent spread towards the lumbar plexus than an infra-inguinal injection: A volunteer study. *Reg Anesth Pain Med.* 2019;44:483-91.

Advancing PENG block techniques for hip analgesia

13

Why this topic is important

Since its introduction in 2018, the pericapsular nerve group (PENG) block has emerged as a motor-sparing regional anesthesia technique for hip analgesia, addressing the need for effective pain control without significant motor blockade. As its adoption has grown, so has our understanding of its anatomical, clinical, and technical considerations.

Objectives of this update

- To summarize the evolution of the PENG block's application and evidence base since its inception.

- To explore the nuances of injectate spread, including desirable and undesirable patterns.

- To review clinical evidence supporting its use for hip fractures, arthroplasty, and other indications.

What is new

Recent studies provide clarity on:

- Optimal injectate volumes to balance analgesic efficacy and motor sparing.

- Patterns of injectate spread, including unintended femoral nerve involvement.

- Comparative effectiveness against other regional anesthesia techniques, such as the fascia iliaca block (FIB).

Understanding injectate spread

Desirable spread

The PENG block targets the articular branches of the femoral, obturator, and accessory obturator nerves (fig-1). Cadaveric studies demonstrate effective anterior and medial hip capsule coverage with 15-20 mL of injectate. This volume ensures pain control by reaching high and low articular branches of these nerves without consistent femoral nerve involvement.

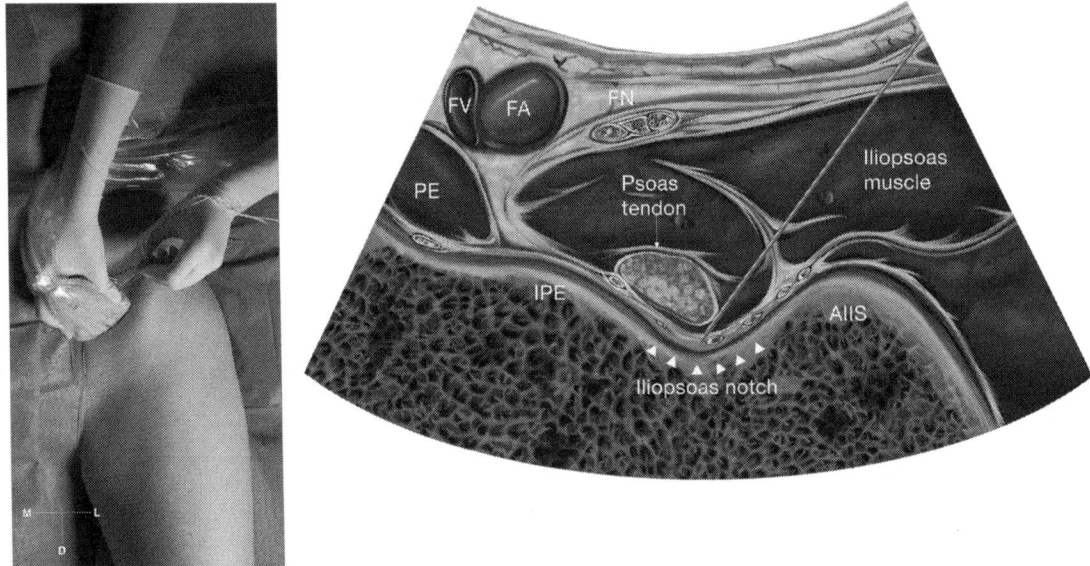

Fig-1. Pericapsular nerve group (PENG) block, reverse ultrasound anatomy. Local anesthetic spread in the plane between the iliopsoas muscle and pubic ramus and the anterior capsule of the hip, thereby anesthetizing the articular branches of the femoral, obturator, and accessory obturator nerves. FA, femoral artery; FV, femoral vein; FN, femoral nerve; PE, pectineus muscle; IPE, iliopubic eminence; AIIS, anterior inferior iliac spine. Image taken from NYSORA LMS. https://nysoralms.com/

Undesirable spread

Increased injectate volumes (e.g., > 20 mL) may lead to unintended spread into:

- The femoral nerve: This occurs alongside the iliopectineal bursa or retrograde migration along the iliopsoas.
- Fascia iliaca compartment: Aberrant spread can result in quadriceps weakness.

Key factors influencing spread include needle placement, patient anatomy, and injection pressure.

Clinical applications and comparative evidence

Alleviating post-traumatic pain in hip fractures

The PENG block is particularly effective for managing dynamic pain after hip fractures, facilitating early mobilization and positioning for spinal anesthesia. Randomized controlled trials (RCTs) demonstrate:

- Significant reductions in dynamic pain scores within hours post-block.

- Improved positioning for spinal anesthesia compared to FIB and sham techniques.

Postoperative analgesia in hip arthroplasty

Multiple RCTs have compared the PENG block with:

1. No block or placebo:
   - Superior pain control and reduced opioid consumption.
   - Faster recovery milestones, including ambulation.

2. Fascia iliaca block:
   - Similar pain control but better quadriceps preservation.
   - Less motor weakness with the PENG block.

Hip arthroscopy and other indications

The PENG block's efficacy is less consistent for hip arthroscopy, likely due to pain sources beyond its sensory coverage. Emerging applications in pediatric surgery and pelvic fractures are promising but require further validation.

Optimizing technique

Injectate volume

The consensus suggests using 15-20 mL to achieve effective analgesia while minimizing femoral nerve involvement. Individualization based on patient anatomy and surgical requirements is critical.

Needle placement

Accurate needle placement lateral to the psoas tendon ensures optimal spread to the targeted nerves. Real-time ultrasound guidance is essential to avoid intramuscular injection or aberrant spread.

Key takeaways

☑ The PENG block provides effective motor-sparing analgesia for hip surgeries, particularly in fracture and arthroplasty cases.

☑ Desirable spread targets articular branches of the femoral, obturator, and accessory obturator nerves, with minimal femoral nerve involvement.

☑ Injectate volumes of 15-20 mL are optimal, balancing pain relief and motor preservation.

☑ Comparative studies favor the PENG block over fascia iliaca blocks for quadriceps preservation and overall recovery outcomes.

☑ Further research must refine its role in hip arthroscopy and newer indications.

Additional recommended reading

1. Girón-Arango L, Peng P. Pericapsular nerve group (PENG) block: what have we learned in the last 5 years? *Reg Anesth Pain Med*. 2024;0:1-8.

2. Balocco AL, Gautier N, Van Boxstael S, et al. Pericapsular nerve group block: a 3D CT scan imaging study to determine the spread of injectate. *Reg Anesth Pain Med*. 2024;0:1-4.

3. Kukreja P, Uppal V, Kofskey AM, et al. Quality of recovery after pericapsular nerve group block for primary total hip arthroplasty under spinal anesthesia: a randomized controlled trial. *Br J Anaesth*. 2023;130:773-779.

Optimal volume for femoral nerve-sparing PENG block

14

Why this topic is important

The pericapsular nerve group (PENG) block, first described in 2018, is increasingly recognized for its motor-sparing properties, particularly in hip surgeries. By selectively targeting the articular branches of the femoral and accessory obturator nerves (fig-1), the PENG block reduces pain while minimizing motor blockade. However, the inadvertent spread of the local anesthetic to the femoral nerve can lead to quadriceps weakness, compromising the block's motor-sparing intent. Optimizing the volume of injectate is crucial to ensuring effective analgesia while preserving muscle function.

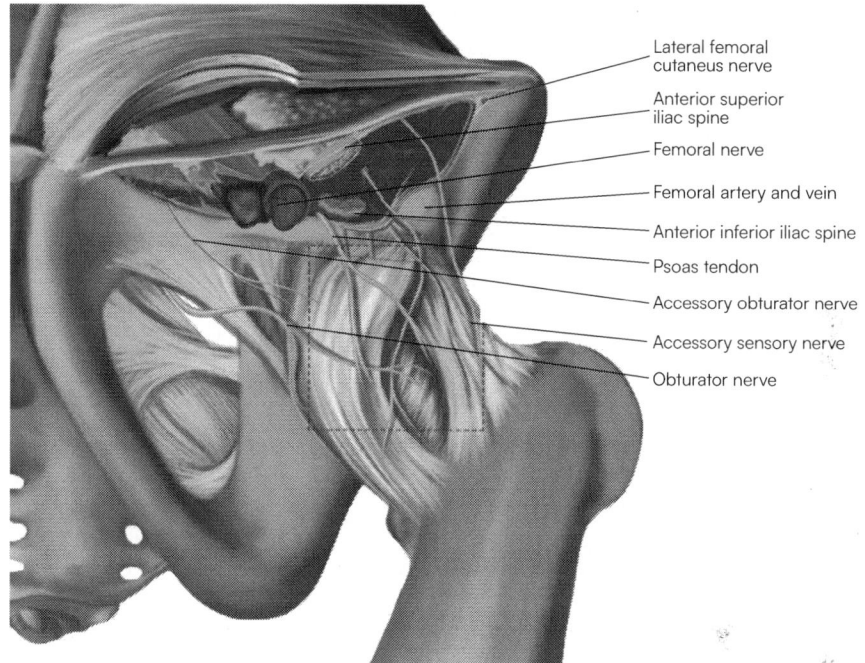

Fig-1. Anterior hip innervantion. Image taken from NYSORA LMS. https://nysoralms.com/

Objectives of this update

- To determine the maximum effective volume (MEV90) of injectate that achieves femoral nerve sparing while effectively targeting the intended articular branches in the PENG block.

- To understand the anatomical patterns of injectate spread and their implications for clinical practice.

- To provide insights for transitioning these findings from a cadaveric model to live patient applications.

What is new

A cadaveric study by Leurcharusmee et al. 2024 is the first to determine the MEV90 for femoral nerve-sparing PENG blocks. The study found that 13.2 mL of methylene blue successfully stained the iliac bone between the anterior inferior iliac spine (AIIS) and iliopubic eminence (IPE) in 90% of cases without staining the femoral nerve.

Findings on femoral nerve-sparing volume

Methodology

- Study design: Cadaveric dose-finding study using the biased coin design method to adjust injectate volume iteratively.

- Sample: 32 cadavers (54 hemipelves).

- Injection technique:

  ○ Ultrasound-guided PENG block targeting the interface between the psoas tendon and the periosteum of the iliac bone.

  ○ Methylene blue was injected at varying volumes to observe its spread and interaction with the femoral nerve.

- Success definition:

  ○ Iliac bone staining between the AIIS and IPE with no femoral nerve staining.

  ○ Any staining of the femoral nerve was deemed a failure.

Key results

1. MEV90 determination

   ○ The MEV90 of methylene blue was 13.2 mL.

   ○ This volume achieved a 93% probability of sparing the femoral nerve while effectively targeting the articular branches.

2. Patterns of dye spread

   ○ Successful blocks exhibited consistent staining of the iliac bone without evidence of dye on the femoral nerve.

   ○ Blocks that failed (femoral nerve stained) showed retrograde spread through the psoas muscle or along its medial margin.

3. Role of needle placement and injection pressure

   ○ Precise needle placement on the iliac bone minimized dye spread toward the femoral nerve.

   ○ Inadequate needle positioning or high injection pressures were associated with unintended spread.

Clinical implications

Optimizing injectate volume for motor-sparing analgesia

The findings underscore the critical role of volume optimization in PENG blocks. Administering 13.2 mL balances effective pain control and preservation of motor function. Higher volumes increase the risk of femoral nerve involvement, potentially leading to quadriceps weakness and impaired ambulation.

Importance of technique in block efficacy

The study highlights the necessity of accurate ultrasound-guided needle placement to avoid the injectate's retrograde spread through the psoas muscle. Controlled injection pressure further minimizes the risk of unintended femoral nerve involvement, ensuring the block's motor-sparing properties.

Translating findings to clinical practice

While the cadaveric model provides foundational insights, further research is needed to validate these findings in live patients. The dynamics of tissue resistance, vascular absorption, and local anesthetic diffusion in live subjects may influence the effective volume and require adjustments to the MEV90 identified in this study.

Limitations

- Cadaveric model: Cadaver studies lack the physiological factors of living tissues, such as blood flow and tissue elasticity, which may affect anesthetic spread.

- Surrogate marker: Methylene blue was used as a proxy for local anesthetic, which may not replicate the precise diffusion properties of agents like ropivacaine or bupivacaine.

Key takeaways

☑ The MEV90 for a femoral nerve-sparing PENG block in a cadaveric model is 13.2 mL of methylene blue, achieving a 93% success rate.

☑ Accurate needle placement on the iliac bone and controlled injection techniques are critical to minimizing unintended femoral nerve involvement.

☑ While the findings provide valuable insights, further research in live patients is essential to confirm their clinical applicability.

☑ Optimizing injectate volume can enhance the block's analgesic efficacy while preserving motor function, supporting faster postoperative recovery.

Additional recommended reading

1. Leurcharusmee P, Kantakam P, Intasuwan P, et al. Cadaveric study investigating the femoral nerve-sparing volume for pericapsular nerve group (PENG) block. *Reg Anesth Pain Med.* 2023;48:549-552.

2. Girón-Arango L, Peng PWH, Chin KJ, et al. Pericapsular nerve group (PENG) block for hip fracture. *Reg Anesth Pain Med.* 2018;43:859-863.

3. Aliste J, Layera S, Bravo D, et al. Randomized comparison between pericapsular nerve group (PENG) block and suprainguinal fascia iliaca block for total hip arthroplasty. *Reg Anesth Pain Med.* 2021;46:874-878.

Pericapsular nerve group (PENG) block: Patterns of spread and risk of femoral nerve block

15

Why this topic is important

The pericapsular nerve group (PENG) block is widely used in anesthesia for hip surgeries, particularly for its motor-sparing properties. This block has emerged as an effective technique to manage postoperative pain with less incidence of significant quadriceps weakness, a frequent drawback of other nerve blocks. Despite its increasing use, much of our understanding of its analgesic mechanisms derives from cadaveric studies. Evaluating the spread in living patients is critical for optimizing its application and outcomes.

Objectives of this update

- To review the findings of Balocco et al. 2024 using 3D CT imaging to assess the spread of local anesthetic during a PENG block.

- To clarify the PENG block's mechanism of action in providing hip analgesia.

- To explore how these findings influence clinical practice, including technique optimization and patient outcomes.

What is new

- A recent study by Balocco et al. 2024 utilized 3D CT imaging to provide the first in vivo insights into the spread of local anesthetic following a PENG block (fig-1). The results challenge previously held assumptions based on cadaveric models, offering a nuanced understanding of its analgesic mechanisms and potential limitations.

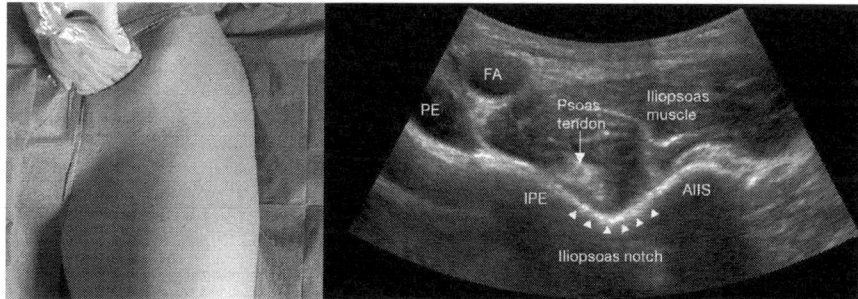

Fig-1. Transducer position and sonoanatomy to perform a hip block. FA, femoral artery; PE, pectineus muscle; IPE, iliopubic eminence; AIIS, anterior inferior iliac spine. Image taken from NYSORA LMS. https://nysoralms.com/

Findings from the 3D CT imaging study

Methodology

Ten patients undergoing hip surgery received an ultrasound-guided PENG block using 18 mL of 0.5% ropivacaine mixed with 2 mL of contrast dye. The injectate spread was assessed using high-resolution CT scans and 3D image reconstructions.

Key results

1. Distribution of injectate

   ◦ The local anesthetic was predominantly confined to the epimysium of the iliacus and psoas muscles.

   ◦ Craneal (pelvic) spread was observed in all patients.

   ◦ Minor spread to the hip capsule was observed, with no evidence of injectate reaching the obturator foramen or subpectineal plane.

2. Implications for the analgesic mechanism

   ◦ The analgesic effect appears primarily related to blocking branches of the femoral nerve within the iliopsoas muscle without reaching the obturator nerve.

   ◦ This distribution suggests the motor-sparing effect may be less reliable in certain patient populations.

3. Comparison with cadaveric studies

   ◦ The live patient study revealed a different effect than cadaveric findings, demonstrating a broader spread to nerves innervating the hip capsule.

   ◦ Tissue characteristics and physiological conditions in living patients likely contribute to these differences.

4. Clinical observations

   ◦ Despite the limited spread, patients reported satisfactory analgesia (pain scores < 3 in the PACU).

◦ The injectate volume and precise needle placement were pivotal in achieving effective outcomes.

Clinical implications

Technique optimization

The study highlights the importance of accurate needle placement; rotating the needle after contacting the bone may enhance the spread within the iliopsoas fascia, achieving the desired analgesic effect. The injected volume could be related to the motor-sparing effects of the block.

Limitations in current understanding

While effective in reducing postoperative pain, the PENG block's inability to consistently block the obturator nerve may limit its use in surgeries requiring broader sensory blockade. Further research is needed to refine the injection technique, volumes required, and patient-specific responses.

Recommendations for practice

- Use real-time ultrasound guidance to ensure anatomical landmark identification and proper needle placement.

- Consider individual patient anatomy and surgical needs when choosing the PENG block.

- Consider adjusting the volume to administer if motor sparing block needs to be secured.

- Evaluate alternative or adjunctive techniques for patients requiring broader nerve coverage.

Key takeaways

☑ The PENG block is a motor-sparing analgesia technique with a probably localized action on the femoral nerve branches within the iliopsoas muscle.

☑ 3D CT imaging in living patients revealed limited spread to the obturator nerve and hip capsule compared to cadaveric studies.

☑ Accurate needle placement and injectate volume are critical to the block's success.

☑ While effective for hip surgeries, the PENG block's limitations warrant further research for broader clinical applications.

Additional recommended reading

1. Balocco AL, Gautier N, Van Boxstael S, et al. Pericapsular nerve group block: a 3D CT scan imaging study to determine the spread of injectate. *Reg Anesth Pain Med.* 2024;0:1-4.

2. Girón-Arango L, Peng PWH, Chin KJ, et al. Pericapsular nerve group (PENG) block for hip fracture. *Reg Anesth Pain Med.* 2018;43(8):859-863.

3. Ahiskalioglu A, Aydin ME, Celik M, et al. Can high volume pericapsular nerve group (PENG) block act as a lumbar plexus block? *J Clin Anesth.* 2020;61:109650.

Adductor canal block techniques: Injectate spread, sciatic nerve involvement, and clinical implications

16

Why this topic is important

Adductor canal blocks (ACBs) are increasingly used for knee surgeries, particularly total knee arthroplasty (TKA), as they provide effective analgesia while sparing quadriceps motor function (fig-1). Despite their advantages, concerns remain about the potential for injectate to spread beyond the adductor canal, especially into the popliteal fossa, where sciatic nerve branches could be inadvertently affected. Such involvement could compromise the technique's motor-sparing benefits and lead to complications like postoperative falls. The cadaveric study of Smulders et al. 2024 investigates whether different ACB techniques and volumes result in sciatic nerve involvement and assesses the extent of injectate spread in distal anatomical regions.

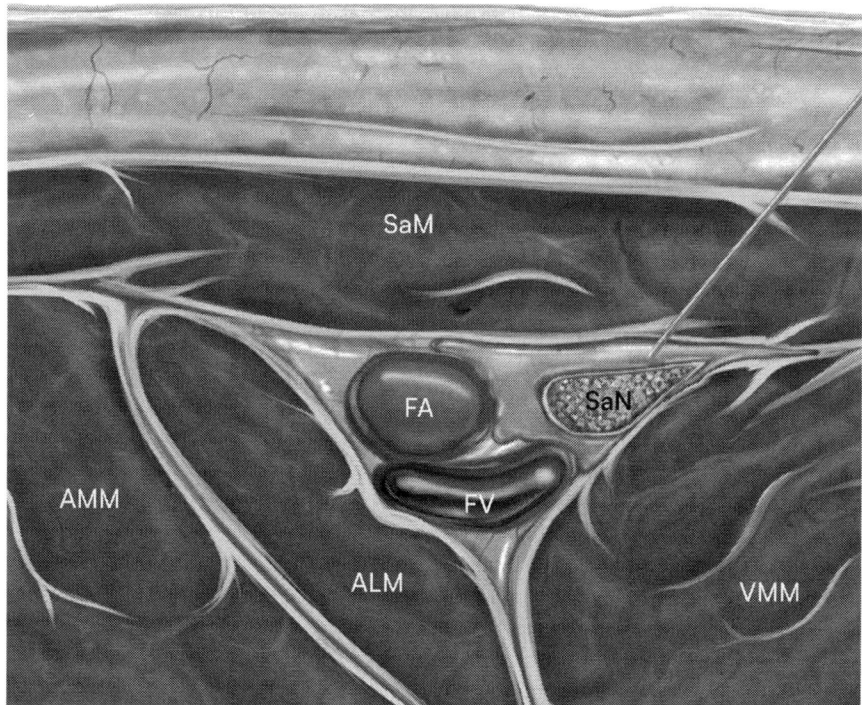

Fig-1. Reverse ultrasound anatomy: Needle insertion and local anesthetic distribution to block the saphenous nerve in the adductor canal. SaN, saphenous nerve; FA, femoral artery; FV, femoral vein; SaM, sartorius muscle; VMM, vastus medialis muscle; ALM, adductor longus muscle.
Image taken from NYSORA LMS. https://nysoralms.com/

Objectives of this update

- To evaluate the incidence of sciatic nerve involvement in various ACB techniques.

- To assess the spread of injectate to the popliteal fossa and its potential implications for clinical practice.

- To explore the efficacy of low- and high-volume injection techniques in achieving targeted analgesia.

What is new

This study by Smulders et al. 2024, using radiological analysis on cadavers, shows that ACB techniques are highly unlikely to involve the sciatic nerve or its branches, even with high injectate volumes. Injectate reached the popliteal fossa in less than 10% of cases, and no adverse effects related to sciatic nerve involvement were noted.

Study findings

Methodology

- Design: Radiological cadaveric study with randomized injection techniques.

- Participants: 18 fresh, unfrozen, and un-embalmed cadavers.

- Techniques:

  - Four ACB variations: mid-thigh (distal femoral triangle) and distal adductor canal, with both low (2 mL) and high (30 mL) injectate volumes.

  - All injections used a 1:10 dilution of contrast medium in local anesthetic.

- Primary outcome: Sciatic nerve involvement, assessed via CT imaging.

- Secondary outcomes: Spread to the popliteal fossa, saphenous nerve coverage, and femoral nerve involvement.

Results

1. Sciatic nerve involvement

   - In any of the 36 blocks performed, no sciatic nerve or branch involvement (tibial or common peroneal nerves) was observed.

2. Injectate spread to the popliteal fossa

   - Spread to the popliteal fossa occurred in only 3 out of 36 injections (8.3%).

   - These cases involved high-volume injections (30 mL) at the distal femoral triangle or distal adductor canal.

3. Saphenous and femoral nerve involvement

   - The saphenous nerve, the primary target of the ACB, was reached in all blocks.

   - The femoral nerve was spared in all injections, confirming the motor-sparing nature of the techniques.

4. Efficacy across techniques

   - In most cases, all techniques successfully confined the injectate to the adductor canal or distal femoral triangle.

   - No differences in injectate spread patterns were attributable to technique or injection site variations.

Clinical implications

Safety of high-volume injections

High-volume ACBs (30 mL) do not involve the sciatic nerve, supporting their use in clinical practice. However, the occasional spread to the popliteal fossa warrants further investigation to determine whether this contributes to enhanced analgesia or presents a risk for unintended motor blockade.

Motor-sparing advantages

Importantly, the study confirms that even with higher-volume injections (30 mL), the injectate does not spread into the femoral triangle, where the femoral nerve supplies the quadriceps. This absence of spread to the femoral triangle is clinically significant because it ensures that quadriceps motor function is preserved, reducing the risk of postoperative falls. Unlike femoral nerve blocks, which can impair quadriceps strength and increase fall risk, ACBs maintain motor function in the quadriceps, making them a safer alternative for TKA and other knee surgeries.

Implications for injectate optimization

Low-volume injections (2 mL) effectively target the saphenous nerve while minimizing the risk of excessive spread. This approach may be suitable for patients at higher risk of complications from larger volumes.

Limitations

- Cadaveric model: Differences between cadaveric and in vivo tissues, such as flow dynamics and tissue elasticity, may affect injectate spread.

- Sample size: Although relatively large for a cadaver study, anatomical variability may still influence results.

- Injection pressure: Injection speed and pressure were not standardized, which could impact injectate spread.

Key takeaways

☑ ACB techniques do not involve the sciatic nerve or its branches, even with high-volume injections (30 mL).

☑ Injectate reaches the popliteal fossa in a minority of cases, but its clinical relevance is unclear.

☑ Saphenous nerve coverage was achieved in all injections, confirming the efficacy of ACBs in targeting knee joint innervation.

☑ ACBs remain a motor-sparing alternative to femoral nerve blocks, reducing the risk of postoperative falls.

Additional recommended reading

1. Smulders PSH, ten Hoope W, Baumann HM, et al. Adductor canal block techniques do not lead to involvement of sciatic nerve branches: a radiological cadaveric study. *Reg Anesth Pain Med.* 2024;49:174-178.

2. Vora MU, Nicholas TA, Kassel CA, et al. Adductor canal block for knee surgical procedures: review article. *J Clin Anesth.* 2016;35:295-303.

3. Gautier PE, Lecoq JP, Hadzic A, et al. Distribution of injectate and sensory-motor blockade after adductor canal block. *Anesth Analg.* 2016;122:279-82.

Popliteal plexus block combined with femoral triangle block after TKA

17

Why this topic is important

Total knee arthroplasty (TKA) is a common orthopedic procedure associated with significant postoperative pain, which can delay mobilization and recovery. Effective pain management strategies that minimize opioid consumption while preserving motor function are crucial for optimizing patient outcomes. Multimodal analgesic protocols incorporating peripheral nerve blocks, such as the adductor canal block (ACB) and femoral triangle block (FTB), have been widely adopted (fig-1).

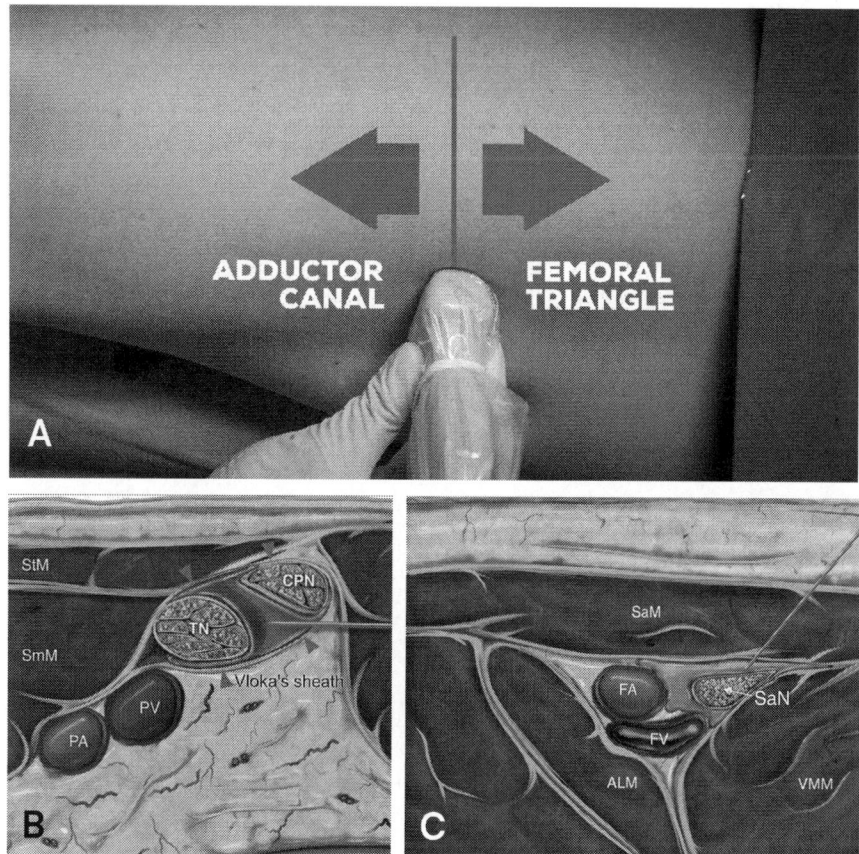

Fig-1A. The femoral triangle is more proximal and contains the proximal saphenous nerve, often a branch to the vastus medialis and sometimes to the obturator nerve, all contributing innervation to the knee joint. The adductor canal contains the distal saphenous nerve, often with the medial femoral cutaneous nerve, and may convey injections into the popliteal fossa.
Fig-1B. Reverse ultrasound anatomy with needle insertion in-plane and local anesthetic distribution to block the sciatic nerve in the popliteal fossa. TN, tibial nerve; CPN, common peroneal nerve; PV, popliteal vein; PA, popliteal artery; StM, semitendinosus muscle; SmM, semimembranosus muscle.
Fig-1C. Reverse ultrasound anatomy, needle insertion, and local anesthetic distribution to block the saphenous nerve in the adductor canal for a femoral triangle block. SaN, saphenous nerve; FA, femoral artery; FV, femoral vein; SaM, sartorius muscle; VMM, vastus medialis muscle; ALM, adductor longus muscle.

Images taken from NYSORA LMS. https://nysoralms.com/

These motor-sparing blocks primarily target sensory innervation to reduce pain without impairing quadriceps strength, facilitating early rehabilitation. The popliteal plexus block (PPB), a novel technique targeting sensory nerves in the posterior knee joint, has shown promise as an adjunct to these established methods. A recent study by Sørensen et al. evaluates the analgesic and functional outcomes of combining PPB with FTB, comparing it to standalone FTB and ACB after TKA.

Objectives of this update

- To assess whether adding PPB to FTB reduces opioid consumption after TKA.
- To examine the impact of PPB on postoperative pain, motor function, and mobilization.
- To explore the potential for PPB to become a standard component of multimodal analgesia protocols.

What is new

This randomized controlled trial by Sørensen et al. 2024 provides the first evidence that adding PPB to FTB significantly reduces 24-hour opioid consumption after TKA without compromising motor function or mobilization.

Study findings

Methodology

- Design: Single-center, triple-arm, randomized controlled trial.
- Participants: 165 adults undergoing primary unilateral TKA with spinal anesthesia.
- Interventions:
  - PPB + FTB group: Received active PPB and FTB with a sham ACB.
  - FTB group: Received active FTB with sham PPB and ACB.
  - ACB group: Received active ACB with sham PPB and FTB.

- Outcomes:
  - Primary: 24-hour postoperative opioid consumption (intravenous oxycodone).
  - Secondary: Pain scores, maximum voluntary isometric contraction (MVIC), timed-up-and-go (TUG) test, and adverse events.

Results

1. Opioid consumption
   - The PPB + FTB group showed significantly lower 24-hour opioid use (median 6 mg) compared to FTB (10 mg) and ACB (12 mg).
   - At 24 hours, 23% of patients in the PPB + FTB group were opioid-free, compared to 11% in the ACB group and 4% in the FTB group.

2. Pain scores
   - Pain scores at rest and during active knee flexion were comparable across all groups and consistently below clinical benchmarks for moderate pain (NRS ≤3 for rest and ≤5 for activity).

3. Motor function
   - MVIC and manual muscle test scores demonstrated no significant differences in knee or ankle strength across groups, confirming that PPB did not impair lower limb motor function.

4. Mobilization
   - All groups achieved similar TUG test times, indicating equivalent ambulation capabilities within the first 24 hours.

5. Safety and adverse events
   - No serious motor deficits were observed, and adverse events were rare. Minor side effects, such as nausea, were similar across groups.

Clinical implications

Enhanced opioid-sparing analgesia

Adding PPB to FTB significantly reduces postoperative opioid consumption without additional risk of motor impairment. This aligns with current efforts to minimize opioid exposure and its associated side effects, particularly in high-risk or opioid-sensitive populations.

Maintenance of motor function and mobilization

The study highlights the safety of PPB as an adjunct to FTB. It preserves the motor-sparing benefits of FTB and ACB, ensuring early rehabilitation and reducing the risk of postoperative complications, such as falls.

Potential standardization in TKA protocols

Incorporating PPB into multimodal analgesia regimens offers a simple and effective way to enhance pain control while supporting functional recovery. This approach may be particularly beneficial in outpatient or fast-track TKA settings where rapid mobilization is a priority.

Limitations

- Single-center design: Results may not generalize to other populations or surgical practices.

- Short-term outcomes: The study focused on 24-hour outcomes, leaving long-term analgesic and functional benefits unexplored.

- Blinding challenges: Sham blocks mimicked the procedures but could not fully replicate the sensation of an active block.

Key takeaways

☑ Adding PPB to FTB significantly reduces 24-hour postoperative opioid consumption compared to standalone FTB or ACB after TKA.

☑ Pain scores were similar across all groups, suggesting that opioid reduction did not compromise pain control.

☑ PPB does not impair motor function or delay mobilization, supporting its role in motor-sparing analgesia strategies.

☑ These findings support the integration of PPB into multimodal analgesia protocols for TKA, although further research is needed to confirm long-term benefits and cost-effectiveness.

Additional recommended reading

1. Sørensen JK, Grevstad U, Jaeger P, et al. Effects of popliteal plexus block after total knee arthroplasty: a randomized clinical trial. *Reg Anesth Pain Med.* 2024;0:1-7.

2. Runge C, Bjørn S, Jensen JM, et al. The analgesic effect of a popliteal plexus blockade after total knee arthroplasty: A feasibility study. *Acta Anaesthesiol Scand.* 2018;62:1127-32.

3. Lavand'homme PM, Kehlet H, Rawal N, et al. Pain management after total knee arthroplasty: procedure-specific postoperative pain management recommendations. *Eur J Anaesthesiol.* 2022;39:743-57.

IPACK blocks in acute pain management after total knee replacement

18

Why this topic is important

Postoperative pain after total knee replacement (TKR) remains a significant challenge, often impairing recovery and patient satisfaction. While adductor canal blocks (ACBs) have become a cornerstone for TKR pain management due to their motor-sparing benefits, they fail to address posterior knee pain, which is innervated by branches of the sciatic nerve.

The introduction of the interspace between the popliteal artery and the capsule of the posterior knee (IPACK) block aims to fill this gap (fig-1). By targeting the posterior capsule of the knee, the IPACK block complements ACBs, offering a comprehensive approach to pain management without impairing motor function. This review evaluates the efficacy of IPACK blocks in combination with ACBs and compares them to alternative analgesic strategies for TKR.

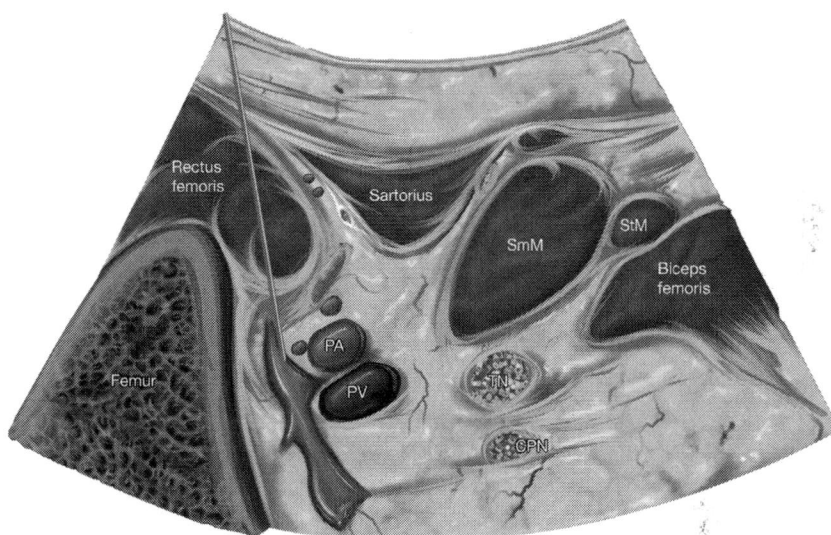

Fig-1. IPACK block, reverse ultrasound anatomy. SmM, semimembranosus muscle; StM, semitendinosus muscle; PA, popliteal artery; PV, popliteal vein; TN, tibial nerve; CPN, common peroneal nerve. Image taken from NYSORA LMS. https://nysoralms.com/

Objectives of this update

- To understand the role of IPACK blocks in addressing posterior knee pain after TKR.

- To evaluate clinical evidence comparing IPACK + ACB to other nerve block combinations and analgesic techniques.

- To explore the risks, benefits, and clinical applications of the IPACK block.

What is new

Recent clinical trials highlight that the IPACK + ACB combination provides superior pain control, reduced opioid consumption, and faster mobilization compared to ACBs alone or other nerve block techniques in many cases. However, conflicting evidence underscores the need for further research.

Findings from clinical trials

Pain relief and opioid consumption

- Studies consistently show that the IPACK + ACB combination significantly reduces pain at rest and during movement in the immediate postoperative period compared to ACB alone or alternative blocks like the sensory posterior articular nerves of the knee (SPANK) block or periarticular multimodal drug injection (PMDI).

- Opioid consumption is generally lower in the IPACK + ACB groups.

- For example, in one study, patients in the IPACK + ACB group required fewer opioids and reported longer times to rescue analgesia compared to the SPANK + ACB group.

Early mobilization

- Multiple studies consistently found that faster mobilization benefited the IPACK + ACB group.

- A randomized trial found that patients receiving IPACK + ACB had quicker ambulation times than those receiving periarticular infiltration (PAI) with ACB or ACB alone.

Conflicting evidence

- Not all studies favor IPACK + ACB.

- Some trials, such as those comparing the IPACK + ACB combination to continuous adductor canal blocks (CACBs), found CACBs to provide superior analgesia and functional outcomes, including better knee flexion and reduced opioid use.

Hospital stays and patient satisfaction

- Hospital stay durations were often comparable between IPACK + ACB and other techniques, though IPACK + ACB was associated with higher patient satisfaction due to effective pain relief and reduced opioid reliance.

Risks and challenges

While the IPACK block is generally considered safe when performed correctly, it carries inherent risks:

- Vascular injury: Proximity to the popliteal artery and vein increases the risk of vascular damage and bleeding.

- Nerve damage: Incorrect needle placement can block the common fibular nerve instead of posterior knee branches, leading to unintended motor deficits.

- Systemic toxicity: Improper injectate placement into systemic circulation may result in arrhythmias, hypotension, or central nervous system effects.

Clinical implications

Integration into multimodal analgesia

- The IPACK block is a valuable addition to multimodal analgesia protocols, complementing ACB to achieve comprehensive pain relief for TKR.

- This combination allows for reduced opioid consumption, enhancing recovery and minimizing opioid-related side effects such as nausea and sedation.

Technique optimization

- Proper needle placement using ultrasound guidance is critical to avoid complications and ensure effective analgesia. Identifying key landmarks, such as the popliteal artery, is essential for successful block execution.

Patient selection

- Patients with high baseline posterior knee pain or a history of poor pain control with ACB alone are ideal candidates for IPACK blocks.

Limitations

- Heterogeneity in study design, including varying techniques, local anesthetic volumes, and concentrations, complicates direct comparisons.

- Long-term outcomes of IPACK + ACB combinations, such as their impact on chronic pain development, remain unclear.

Key takeaways

- ☑ IPACK blocks effectively complement ACBs in addressing posterior knee pain after TKR, offering superior pain relief and reduced opioid consumption compared to ACBs alone or other techniques.

- ☑ Faster mobilization and higher patient satisfaction are significant benefits of the IPACK + ACB combination.

- ☑ While generally safe, the IPACK block requires precise technique and proper patient selection to maximize benefits and minimize risks.

Additional recommended reading

1. Upshaw WC, Richey JM, Tassin JP, et al. IPACK Block Efficacy for Acute Pain Management after Total Knee Replacement: A Review. *Curr Pain Headache Rep.* 2024;28:673-679.

2. Guo J, Hou M, Shi G, et al. iPACK block added to adductor canal blocks versus the adductor canal blocks in pain management after total knee arthroplasty: A systematic review and meta-analysis. *J Orthop Surg Res.* 2022;17(1):387.

3. Tang X, Jiang X, Lei L, et al. IPACK block combined with single adductor canal block versus single adductor canal block for analgesia after total knee arthroplasty. *Orthop Surg.* 2022;14(11):2809-21.

Distal subsartorial compartment block of the saphenous nerve

19

Why this topic is important

Effective post-surgical analgesia, especially in foot and ankle procedures, is critical given the substantial pain these surgeries often generate. One commonly used intervention is the saphenous nerve block, as this nerve innervates the anteromedial regions of the foot and ankle, which are major sources of post-surgical pain. Traditionally, saphenous nerve blocks are performed in the femoral triangle, which, although effective, often leads to unwanted quadriceps motor impairment, thus limiting early postoperative mobility.

To improve patient outcomes, there is a growing need to refine regional anesthesia techniques that can provide sufficient analgesia without affecting motor function. The distal subsartorial compartment block (DSCB) offers a promising alternative. By targeting the saphenous nerve after it exits the adductor canal, the DSCB provides effective sensory blockade with minimal risk of quadriceps impairment. This technique has great potential to enhance post-surgical recovery, reduce opioid reliance, and improve overall patient satisfaction.

Objectives of this update

- To review the anatomical background and clinical relevance of the distal subsartorial compartment block (DSCB)

- To outline step-by-step procedural techniques for safely targeting the saphenous nerve using ultrasound guidance

- To evaluate findings from cadaveric dissections and clinical case series to assess the effectiveness of DSCB in foot and ankle surgery

What is new

A recent study by Jensen et al.[1] introduces a refined method for selectively anesthetizing the saphenous nerve in the distal subsartorial compartment. Cadaveric dissections demonstrate that this approach effectively anesthetizes the saphenous nerve with a high degree of specificity, sparing quadriceps motor function in all cases but two (13%). Findings from a clinical case series confirm the procedure's effectiveness, with all patients reporting complete sensory blockade in the targeted areas and full ambulatory ability post-surgery. The innovative use of AI-enhanced MRI further elucidates the nerve's path, aiding clinicians in accurately identifying landmarks essential for successful blockade.

Anatomy and relevance of the saphenous nerve

The saphenous nerve, a branch of the femoral nerve, provides sensory innervation to the anteromedial aspect of the lower leg, ankle, and foot. It exits the adductor canal distally, continuing along the medial thigh and leg, eventually becoming superficial between the tendons of the sartorius and gracilis muscles.

Given its course and distribution, the saphenous nerve block is frequently employed for surgeries involving the foot and ankle. However, a femoral triangle block for the saphenous nerve often causes quadriceps weakness by inadvertently anesthetizing motor branches of the femoral nerve, such as the medial vastus nerve. This quadriceps impairment limits mobility, presenting challenges in early recovery.

A true adductor canal block offers some motor-sparing advantages over the femoral triangle approach, but research has shown that it, too, may lead to quadriceps weakness due to proximal anesthetic spread. In contrast, DSCB targets the saphenous nerve distal to the adductor canal and avoids proximal spread, ensuring effective sensory blockade without affecting quadriceps strength. This characteristic makes it ideal for foot and ankle surgeries where early ambulation is critical.

Procedural technique: Ultrasound-guided distal subsartorial compartment block

Patient positioning:

To perform the DSCB, position the patient supine with slight external thigh rotation and mild knee flexion.

Ultrasound setup:

Use a high-frequency linear probe (15 MHz) to identify the sartorius muscle approximately at the level of the patella's base. Once located, follow the sartorius muscle proximally and distally until the segment where the saphenous nerve intersects with the tendon of the adductor magnus muscle can be identified.

Needle placement and anesthetic injection:

With ultrasound guidance, insert the needle in-plane from an anterior approach and direct it to the subsartorial compartment, where the saphenous nerve can be visualized distal to the adductor canal. A 5-10 ml volume of anesthetic is typically sufficient to anesthetize the nerve without affecting nearby structures.

The procedure's ease and high success rate, demonstrated in both cadaveric studies and clinical cases, suggest its applicability in diverse clinical settings. Additionally, it allows for reliable, effective, and quick application, with typical completion time averaging about 1 minute and 20 seconds.

Dissection study findings

A dissection study was conducted using 15 cadaveric sides to assess the accuracy and specificity of the DSCB. The technique was successful in targeting the saphenous nerve, as evidenced by selective staining with methylene blue:

- Success rate: In all 15 specimens, the saphenous nerve was stained, confirming effective anesthetic targeting.

- Motor-sparing effect: Only two out of 15 cadaveric specimens (13%) showed incidental staining of the medial vastus nerve, meaning that DSCB avoids clinically significant quadriceps impairment.

The low incidence of medial vastus nerve involvement underscores the motor-sparing effect of DSCB, making it advantageous over proximal techniques that increase the risk of quadriceps weakness.

Clinical case series results

A clinical case series of five patients was conducted to validate the clinical applicability and effectiveness of the DSCB for postoperative pain management in foot and ankle surgeries:

- Block effectiveness: All five patients experienced complete sensory anesthesia in the targeted anteromedial area of the lower leg, with a 100% success rate in achieving a cutaneous area of anesthesia.

- Mobility outcomes: Each patient retained full ambulatory capacity without any support post-surgery, reinforcing the motor-sparing nature of DSCB. Quadriceps strength was preserved, and no patients reported weakness in the operated limb.

- Analgesic efficacy: Postoperative pain scores were uniformly low (NRS score 0) in the saphenous nerve distribution area, demonstrating effective analgesia.

These results indicate that DSCB offers robust pain control, enhances patient comfort, and allows for immediate postoperative ambulation. One patient reported some pain in the dorsum of the foot and lateral ankle, which was resolved with a supplemental sciatic nerve block.

Insights from AI-enhanced MRI imaging

An innovative addition to this study was the use of ai-enhanced MRI, which provided high-resolution visualization of the saphenous nerve's path from the adductor canal to its emergence in the subsartorial compartment.

- Nerve trajectory: MRI findings showed the saphenous nerve exiting the adductor canal and following a predictable path, allowing practitioners to identify target landmarks for DSCB accurately.

- Medial vastus nerve: The medial vastus nerve was consistently found outside the adductor canal in a separate fascial tunnel, reinforcing the anatomical feasibility of motor-sparing blocks.

- Co-anesthetized nerves: The AI-MRIi also identified the proximity of the anterior branch of the medial femoral cutaneous nerve, which lies close to the saphenous nerve. This explains the occasional co-anesthesia observed in the medial thigh region, although it does not affect quadriceps function.

AI-enhanced imaging solidifies the DSCB's anatomic reliability and highlights its effectiveness as a selective, motor-sparing technique. Further research may expand on the use of AI-enhanced MRI for detailed nerve mapping in regional anesthesia.

Clinical advantages and limitations of DSCB

Advantages

- Enhanced mobility: By avoiding quadriceps impairment, DSCB enables patients to ambulate early postoperatively, a key factor in enhanced recovery protocols for foot and ankle surgery.

- Reduced opioid requirements: Effective peripheral nerve block techniques, like DSCB, reduce the need for opioids and their associated side effects.

- High success rate: DSCB is highly reliable and has a 100% success rate in both dissection and clinical cases, making it a valuable technique for anesthesiologists.

Limitations

- Technical skill requirement: While relatively simple, the DSCB requires ultrasound-guided precision. Challenges may arise in patients with subcutaneous edema or high BMI, where visualization can be impaired.

- Need for further clinical validation: This technique was studied on a limited sample size of five clinical cases. Larger-scale studies are needed to fully validate the clinical benefits of DSCB across diverse populations and settings.

Key takeaways

☑ The distal subsartorial compartment block (DSCB) selectively anesthetizes the saphenous nerve without impacting quadriceps function, making it ideal for foot and ankle surgeries.

☑ Ultrasound guidance is key to effectively performing DSCB and achieving high success rates with minimal risk of motor impairment.

☑ Patient case series show DSCB's effectiveness in reducing postoperative pain and maintaining ambulation, with high patient satisfaction.

☑ Ai-enhanced MRI provides critical anatomical insights, confirming the nerve's course and reinforcing dscb's motor-sparing nature.

Additional recommended reading

1. Jensen AE, Bjørn S, Nielsen TD, et al. Distal subsartorial compartment block of the saphenous nerve: A dissection study and a patient case series. *J Clin Anesth.* 2024;92:111315.

2. Bjørn S, Wong YY, Baas J, et al. The importance of the saphenous nerve block for analgesia following major ankle surgery: A randomized, controlled, double-blind study. *Reg Anesth Pain Med.* 2018;43:474-9.

3. Van Der Wal M, Lang SA, Yip RW. Transsartorial approach for saphenous nerve block. *Can J Anaesth.* 1993;40:542-6.

The efficacy of plantar compartment block for postoperative analgesia in hallux valgus surgery

20

Why this topic is important

Hallux valgus surgery, commonly known as bunion surgery, is often performed in outpatient settings and is associated with significant postoperative pain. Effective analgesia following this surgery is crucial, as patients typically want to resume normal ambulation quickly. Standard analgesic techniques, such as the popliteal sciatic nerve block (PSNB, fig-1) and ankle blocks (fig-2), are frequently used for these procedures but have drawbacks. These include impairing proprioception and heel sensitivity, which are vital for safe ambulation. Proprioceptive impairment can increase the risk of falls, especially in outpatient settings where patients are expected to mobilize independently post-surgery.

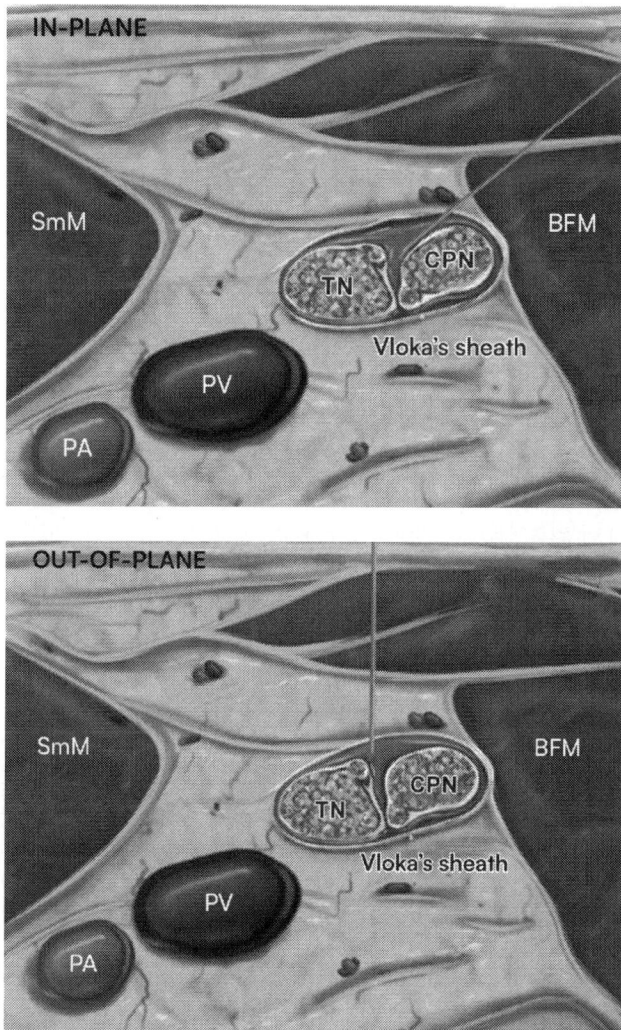

Fig-1. Reverse ultrasound anatomy of local anesthetic spread surrounding the sciatic nerve within Vloka's sheath using an in-plane (top) or out-of-plane (bottom) approach to the popliteal sciatic nerve block. CPN, Common peroneal nerve; PV Popliteal vein; PA, Popliteal artery; SmM, Semimembranosus muscle; BFM, biceps femoris muscle.
Image taken from NYSORA LMS. https://nysoralms.com/

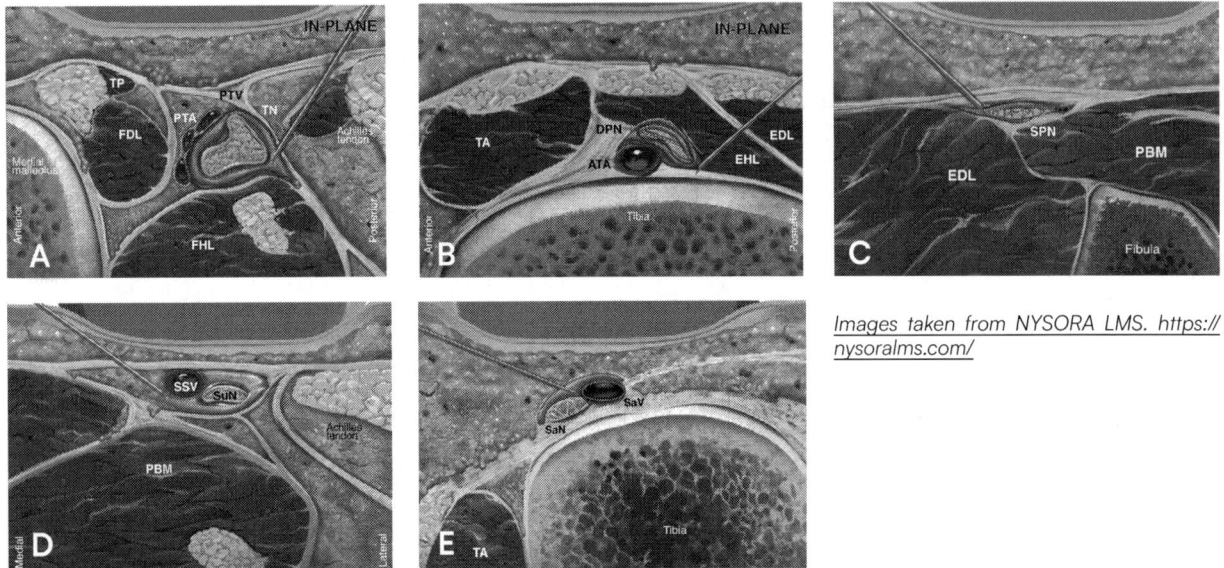

Fig-2A. Reverse ultrasound anatomy of a tibial nerve block with needle insertion in-plane. TP, tibialis posterior muscle; FDL, flexor digitorum longus; PTA, posterior tibial artery; PTV, posterior tibial vein; TN, tibial nerve; FHL, flexor hallucis longus. Fig-2B. Reverse ultrasound anatomy of a deep peroneal nerve block with needle insertion in-plane. TA, tibialis anterior; ATA, anterior tibial artery (also called "Dorsalis Pedis Artery"); DPN, deep peroneal nerve; EHL, extensor hallucis longus, EDL, extensor digitorum longus. Fig-2C. Reverse ultrasound anatomy of a superficial peroneal nerve block with needle insertion in-plane. EDL, extensor digitorum longus; SPN, superficial peroneal nerve; PBM, peroneus brevis muscle. Fig-2D. Reverse ultrasound anatomy of a sural nerve block with needle insertion in-plane. SuN, sural nerve; SSV, small saphenous vein; PBM, peroneus brevis muscle. Fig-2E. Reverse ultrasound anatomy of a saphenous nerve block with needle insertion in-plane. TA, tibialis anterior muscle; SaN, saphenous nerve; SaV, saphenous vein.

The plantar compartment block (PCB) offers a more targeted approach. PCB primarily anesthetizes the medial and lateral plantar nerves responsible for sensation in the forefoot and plantar regions without affecting the heel's proprioceptive function. By preserving heel sensitivity and proprioception, PCB allows for safer postoperative ambulation while providing effective pain control in the operated area. A recent study[1] explores PCB's anatomical feasibility and clinical efficacy, assessing its potential as a safer alternative to PSNB for outpatient hallux valgus surgeries.

Objectives of this update

- Evaluate anatomical feasibility and spread of PCB: Understand the spread patterns of injectate in the plantar compartment, targeting key sensory nerves.

- Assess clinical outcomes: Measure the effectiveness of PCB in managing postoperative pain, time to first analgesic request, and patient mobility.

- Guide technique selection: Provide insights into the advantages of PCB over traditional blocks like PSNB, particularly in enhancing safe ambulation for outpatient hallux valgus surgeries.

What is new

- Selective analgesia with heel sensitivity preservation: PCB effectively blocks the medial and lateral plantar nerves, allowing for targeted pain relief without compromising proprioception, which is essential for safe ambulation.

- Extended pain control duration: PCB using ropivacaine resulted in a median sensory block duration of over 17 hours, providing patients with a prolonged pain-free period post-surgery.

- High patient satisfaction and safety profile: PCB demonstrated high success rates in pain management, reduced opioid use, early ambulation, and minimal side effects, supporting its use for hallux valgus surgery in outpatient settings.

Clinical study overview

Methods

The study included both anatomical and clinical components to explore PCB's applicability for hallux valgus surgery.

1. Anatomical study:

   ◦ Cadaveric dissections were performed to examine the plantar compartment and assess injectate spread to targeted nerve structures.

   ◦ Using 5 mL of colored gelatin injected into the plantar compartment, researchers confirmed that the injectate reliably reached the medial and lateral plantar nerves without affecting structures outside the compartment.

2. Clinical study:

   ◦ Thirty patients undergoing outpatient hallux valgus surgery received a PCB combined with a PSNB for intraoperative anesthesia.

   ◦ The PCB was administered using an ultrasound-guided technique with 5 mL of ropivacaine 0.5%, targeting the medial and lateral plantar nerves. For complete analgesia of the foot, 2.5 mL of ropivacaine was injected near each peroneal nerve.

   ◦ Outcomes measured included sensory block duration, postoperative pain scores via the Visual Analog Scale (VAS), time to first request for rescue analgesics, functional ambulation, and overall patient satisfaction.

Results

1. Anatomical findings:

   ◦ Dissections revealed that a single medial calcaneal nerve branches into the medial and lateral plantar nerves within the plantar compartment. Injecting 5 mL of anesthetic provided effective coverage for these nerves, with minimal extraneous spread.

2. Postoperative pain control and duration of analgesia:

   ◦ The median duration of PCB's sensory block was 17.3 hours, with the first rescue analgesia request occurring at a median of 11.75 hours postoperatively.

   ◦ Pain scores were consistently low, with a median VAS score of 2 or less over the first 48 hours, indicating effective and extended pain control.

3. Functional recovery and ambulation:

   ◦ 90% of patients achieved functional ambulation and discharge criteria within five hours post-surgery. Ambulation criteria included the ability to walk without crutches, maintain heel sensation, and lift the heel from the ground.

   ◦ PCB allowed patients to mobilize safely and independently, preserving proprioception in the heel, a feature particularly beneficial in outpatient surgery where rapid, safe discharge is essential.

4. Patient satisfaction and safety:

   ◦ High patient satisfaction was reported, with 87% of patients expressing complete satisfaction with their postoperative pain management and mobility.

   ◦ No adverse events or complications related to PCB were reported, underscoring its safety and feasibility as an analgesic option in hallux valgus surgeries.

Discussion

Advantages of plantar compartment block in hallux valgus surgery

1. Selective analgesia with preservation of heel proprioception: PCB's ability to anesthetize only the medial and lateral plantar nerves while sparing the heel makes it an optimal choice for procedures requiring effective analgesia without impairing balance or proprioception. This is particularly beneficial for outpatient surgeries, as it reduces the likelihood of falls and allows patients to walk safely and confidently without assistance.

2. Extended pain relief with reduced opioid use: The extended duration of pain relief provided by PCB (over 17 hours on average) minimizes the need for additional analgesics, particularly opioids, in the early postoperative period. This is a significant advantage in reducing postoperative opioid consumption, which can mitigate risks associated with opioid use, such as nausea, sedation, and addiction.

3. Efficient functional recovery supporting outpatient discharge: The rapid recovery and functional mobility achieved with PCB align well with outpatient surgical protocols that prioritize early discharge. Patients demonstrated the ability to perform functional tasks such as heel lifting and unassisted walking within hours after surgery, which is an improvement over traditional blocks like PSNB, where proprioception is often compromised, requiring crutches or assistance.

4. Precision and safety of US-guided PCB: The use of ultrasound guidance in PCB allows for precise anesthetic placement, minimizing the risk of anesthetic spread to non-targeted areas or the need for excessive local anesthetic. The consistency in injectate placement seen in the anatomical study supports ultrasound guidance as a reliable method for administering PCB, ensuring consistent outcomes and reducing the likelihood of unintentional motor block.

Clinical implications and recommendations for practice

1. Indications for using PCB in outpatient forefoot surgery: For hallux valgus and similar forefoot surgeries, PCB is a viable alternative to PSNB, offering comparable analgesia with the added benefit of proprioception preservation. This is particularly advantageous in outpatient settings where early mobilization and safe ambulation are priorities.

2. Combination with peroneal blocks for complete foot analgesia: While PCB covers the plantar aspect effectively, peroneal nerve blocks (superficial and deep) are recommended to achieve complete anesthesia of the foot's dorsal surface. This combination ensures comprehensive pain management for procedures like hallux valgus surgery, as the peroneal nerves provide sensation to the dorsal forefoot.

3. Potential broader applications of PCB: PCB's efficacy and safety profile suggest it could be useful for other foot surgeries requiring plantar analgesia with rapid postoperative ambulation. Procedures involving the forefoot and midfoot, where preserving heel proprioception is desirable, may benefit from PCB as an alternative to more extensive blocks like PSNB.

4. Practical considerations for clinicians:

   ◦ Technique: Accurate ultrasound guidance is essential for effective PCB, as this minimizes extraneous anesthetic spread and preserves proprioception. Clinicians should ensure they are comfortable with ultrasound-guided regional anesthesia techniques.

   ◦ Patient selection: PCB is well-suited for outpatient procedures in patients without contraindications to nerve blocks and who are expected to ambulate soon after surgery. Its suitability extends to patients who may be at increased risk of falls due to proprioceptive loss from other nerve block techniques.

Key takeaways

☑ Selective analgesia promoting ambulation: PCB effectively blocks the medial and lateral plantar nerves while sparing heel sensation, making it ideal for safe postoperative ambulation.

☑ Prolonged analgesia with minimal rescue analgesics: PCB provides a median sensory block duration of over 17 hours, significantly reducing early postoperative opioid requirements.

☑ Efficient for outpatient hallux valgus surgery: The high rate of early mobility and functional discharge makes PCB well-suited for outpatient hallux valgus surgeries.

☑ High patient satisfaction and low adverse event profile: PCB showed excellent patient satisfaction, with no reported adverse events, underscoring its safety and efficacy for outpatient applications.

Additional recommended reading

1. Herteleer, M., Choquet, O., Swisser, F., et al. "Plantar compartment block for hallux valgus surgery: a proof-of-concept anatomic and clinical study." *Reg Anesth Pain Med* 2024.

2. Korwin-Kochanowska, K., Potié, A., El-Boghdadly, K., et al. "PROSPECT guideline for hallux valgus repair surgery: a systematic review and procedure-specific postoperative pain management recommendations." *Reg Anesth Pain Med* 2020;45:702-8.

3. Klein, S. M., Evans, H., Nielsen, K. C., et al. "Peripheral nerve block techniques for ambulatory surgery." *Anesth Analg* 2005;101:1663-76.

Plantar compartment block after hallux valgus surgery

21

Why this topic is important

Hallux valgus surgery is a common outpatient procedure often accompanied by significant postoperative pain and mobility challenges, which can hinder recovery and increase the need for narcotics. Traditional analgesic approaches, such as the popliteal sciatic nerve block (PSNB), effectively control pain but may impair ambulation due to motor and sensory blockades, including heel insensitivity. This limitation raises concerns about fall risk and delays in functional recovery.

The plantar compartment block (PCB) is a novel ultrasound-guided regional anesthesia technique targeting the medial and lateral plantar nerves while sparing the calcaneal branch, preserving heel sensation. This innovative approach may facilitate earlier unassisted walking while providing adequate pain control. Understanding whether PCB can enhance recovery compared to standard techniques like PSNB is essential for improving outcomes in foot surgeries.

Objectives of this update

- To compare the effectiveness of PCB combined with a short-acting PSNB versus a long-acting PSNB alone in enabling unaided walking postoperatively.

- To assess the impact on gait quality, pain relief, and recovery metrics such as opioid consumption and patient satisfaction.

- To evaluate PCB's role in minimizing fall risk and optimizing rehabilitation in outpatient settings.

What is new

A recent study by Swisser et al. 2024 demonstrates that PCB significantly reduces time to unaided ambulation, improves gait quality, and provides effective pain relief compared to PSNB, marking a shift in regional anesthesia strategies for foot surgery recovery.

Key findings

Study design

- Participants: 59 patients undergoing outpatient hallux valgus surgery, randomized to two groups:

  - PCB group: PCB with short-acting PSNB and fibular blocks.

  - Control group: Long-acting PSNB with sham PCB and fibular blocks.

- Primary outcome: Proportion of patients able to walk unaided 6 hours postoperatively.

- Secondary outcomes: Gait quality (assessed using GAITRite), time to free ambulation, opioid use, and patient satisfaction.

Results

1. Ambulation success:

   - 70% of the PCB group achieved unaided walking within 6 hours, compared to 13.8% in the control group.

2. Gait quality:

   - PCB improved Functional Ambulation Profile (FAP) scores (63 vs. 49.5) and reduced gait asymmetry compared to PSNB.

3. Time to free ambulation at home:

   - Median time to unaided walking was 9 hours in the PCB group versus 33.5 hours in the control group.

4. Postoperative analgesia:

   - Pain levels and opioid consumption were comparable between groups, but PCB was associated with earlier pain onset due to its shorter duration of sensory block.

5. Safety:

   - No falls, neuropathies, or serious adverse events were reported in either group.

Clinical implications

Enhanced recovery and mobility

- PCB's ability to preserve heel sensation and improve gait dynamics significantly accelerates ambulation, a critical factor in outpatient recovery.

- Patients receiving PCB are less likely to require crutches or experience postural instability, minimizing the risk of falls and enabling faster functional recovery.

Practical recommendations

- Use PCB in combination with short-acting PSNB for patients undergoing hallux valgus surgery to optimize early mobility and maintain effective pain control.

- Employ ultrasound guidance to ensure accurate nerve targeting and minimize procedural complications.

Limitations and future directions

Study limitations

- The lack of a direct comparison with ankle blocks limits conclusions about PCB's broader applicability.

- The monocentric design may restrict generalizability.

Future research

- Compare PCB directly with other regional techniques, such as ankle blocks, in similar surgical populations.

- Investigate the cost-effectiveness of PCB in enhancing recovery and reducing hospital readmissions.

Key takeaways

☑ PCB facilitates earlier unaided walking and improves gait quality compared to PSNB in patients undergoing hallux valgus surgery.

☑ This novel approach preserves heel sensation, reducing fall risk and enhancing recovery in outpatient settings.

☑ PCB represents a promising addition to multimodal analgesia strategies, combining effective pain relief with functional benefits.

Additional recommended reading

1. Swisser F, Brethe Y, Choquet O, et al. Plantar compartment block improves enhanced recovery after hallux valgus surgery: A randomized, comparative, double-blind study. *Anesthesiology*. 2024;141:891-903.

2. Herteleer M, Choquet O, Swisser F, et al. Plantar compartment block for hallux valgus surgery: A proof-of-concept anatomic and clinical study. *Reg Anesth Pain Med*. 2024 [Epub ahead of print].

3. Olofsson M, Nguyen A, Rossel JB, Albrecht E. Duration of analgesia after forefoot surgery compared between an ankle and a sciatic nerve block at the popliteal crease: A randomized controlled single-blinded trial. *Eur J Anaesthesiol*. 2024;41:55-60.

Efficacy of suprainguinal fascia iliaca block for analgesia after total hip arthroplasty

22

Why this topic is important

Total hip arthroplasty (THA) is associated with significant postoperative pain, which can delay recovery and reduce patient satisfaction. Effective pain management is essential to enhance recovery, minimize opioid consumption, and improve functional outcomes. Regional anesthesia, including the fascia iliaca block, has been proposed as a means of reducing postoperative pain and opioid use. The suprainguinal fascia iliaca block (SIFIB), performed under ultrasound guidance (fig-1), has been suggested as a safer alternative to posterior lumbar plexus blocks due to its simplicity and reduced risk profile. However, its effectiveness in reducing pain and opioid consumption in the context of multimodal analgesia after THA is not well established.

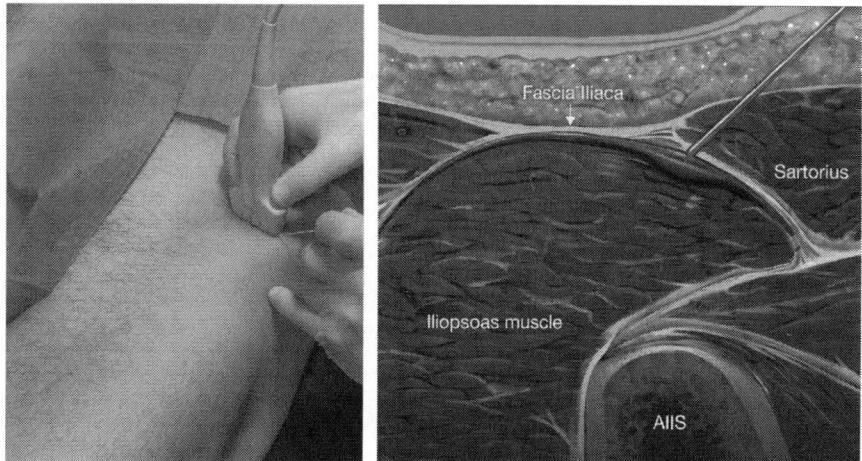

Fig-1. Reverse ultrasound anatomy for a suprainguinal approach to a fascia iliaca block. Needle insertion is shown in-plane with LA distribution (blue) under the fascia iliaca. AIIS, anterior inferior iliac spine. Image taken from NYSORA LMS. https://nysoralms.com/

Objectives of this update

- To assess whether SIFIB reduces postoperative opioid consumption in the first 24 hours after THA.

- To evaluate its impact on secondary outcomes, including pain scores, opioid-related side effects, and functional recovery.

- To determine whether SIFIB enhances early postoperative recovery when added to a multimodal analgesia regimen.

What is new

A recent randomized, placebo-controlled trial by Safa et al.[1] is among the first to rigorously evaluate the impact of SIFIB on opioid consumption and pain outcomes in patients undergoing elective THA under spinal anesthesia.

Key findings

Study design and participants

- Participants: 134 adults aged 18—80 years undergoing elective THA with spinal anesthesia.

- Intervention groups:

  ○ Block group: Ultrasound-guided SIFIB with 40 mL of 0.5% ropivacaine.

  ○ Sham block group: Ultrasound-guided injection of 40 mL of saline.

- Primary outcome: Opioid consumption (oral morphine equivalent, OME) in the first 24 hours postoperatively.

- Secondary outcomes: Pain scores at rest and during movement, opioid-related side effects (e.g., nausea, vomiting, respiratory depression), and the ability to perform physiotherapy.

Results

1. Primary outcome: Opioid consumption

   ○ Mean opioid consumption in the first 24 hours postoperatively was similar between groups, with 63.4 mg OME in the block group and 67.0 mg OME in the sham group.

2. Secondary outcomes

   ○ Pain scores: Within the first 24 hours, no significant differences were observed in pain scores at rest or during movement between the block and sham groups.

   ○ Side effects: Rates of opioid-related side effects, including nausea and vomiting, were comparable between the two groups.

   ○ Physiotherapy participation: Both groups demonstrated similar ability to participate in early postoperative physiotherapy, with no significant differences in mobility or quadriceps weakness.

Clinical implications

Reevaluating SIFIB's role in multimodal analgesia

- Lack of superiority: This study found no evidence that SIFIB with ropivacaine provided significant opioid-sparing or pain-relieving benefits over a sham block when both were used in conjunction with a robust multimodal analgesic regimen.

- Integration in clinical practice: The findings challenge the routine use of SIFIB in THA, suggesting that its benefits may be limited in the context of effective multimodal strategies already in place.

Practical considerations

- Use in specific scenarios: While the study does not support widespread use, SIFIB may still be useful in cases where other multimodal components are contraindicated or unavailable.

- Technique and monitoring: Ensuring block efficacy through proper technique and volume may enhance outcomes in selected patients, particularly in ambulatory or resource-limited settings.

Limitations and future directions

Study limitations

- Block verification: The study did not assess the success of individual blocks, potentially diluting observed effects.

- Population: Findings are limited to patients receiving spinal anesthesia with multimodal analgesia; results may differ in populations with general anesthesia or reduced multimodal options.

Future research

- Investigate SIFIB's efficacy in alternative surgical settings, such as ambulatory THA or anterior hip approaches.

- Explore the impact of higher local anesthetic volumes or alternative agents on block efficacy.

- Evaluate long-term outcomes, such as opioid dependence and functional recovery.

Key takeaways

☑ The addition of SIFIB with ropivacaine to multimodal analgesia did not reduce opioid consumption or pain scores compared to a sham block in the first 24 hours post-THA.

☑ SIFIB's role may be limited in settings where robust multimodal analgesia is employed.

☑ Further studies are needed to refine patient selection and optimize block technique.

Additional recommended reading

1. Safa B, Trinh H, Lansdown A, et al. Ultrasound-guided suprainguinal fascia iliaca compartment block and early postoperative analgesia after total hip arthroplasty: A randomized controlled trial. Br J Anaesth. 2024;133(1):146-151.

2. Desmet M, Vermeylen K, Van Herreweghe I, et al. A longitudinal suprainguinal fascia iliaca compartment block reduces morphine consumption after total hip arthroplasty. Reg Anesth Pain Med. 2017;42(3):327-33.

3. Gasanova I, Alexander JC, Estrera K, et al. Ultrasound-guided suprainguinal fascia iliaca compartment block versus periarticular infiltration for pain management after total hip arthroplasty: A randomized controlled trial. Reg Anesth Pain Med. 2019;44(2):206-211.

Regional anesthesia in specific surgeries

Regional or general anesthesia for total joint arthroplasty

23

Why this topic is important

Total joint arthroplasty (TJA) for hips and knees is one of the most effective treatments for advanced osteoarthritis, offering significant improvements in pain relief, joint function, and overall quality of life. As the global population ages, the number of TJAs performed annually increases exponentially, making this procedure a public health priority. In the United States alone, demand for total hip arthroplasty (THA) and total knee arthroplasty (TKA) is projected to increase by 174% and 673% by 2030, respectively.

Given the scale of these surgeries, selecting the optimal anesthesia technique-regional anesthesia (RA) versus general anesthesia (GA-has important implications for patient outcomes. RA, which includes spinal or epidural anesthesia, offers potential benefits over GA, such as fewer intubation complications and reduced respiratory issues risks. Yet, findings on the impact of RA versus GA on mortality and postoperative complications have been inconsistent, with some studies favoring RA for reducing mortality but failing to show clear superiority in terms of complications. This update, based on a recent nationwide cohort study from South Korea[1], provides valuable insights into these two anesthesia techniques, helping clinicians make more informed choices when managing patients undergoing TJA.

Objectives of this update

- Review the impact of regional anesthesia (RA) versus general anesthesia (GA) on 30-day and 90-day postoperative mortality in patients undergoing total hip or knee arthroplasty.

- Examine whether RA offers advantages in reducing the rate of postoperative complications compared to GA.

- Highlight differences in anesthesia outcomes between total hip arthroplasty (THA) and total knee arthroplasty (TKA).

- Provide clinical guidance on the selection of anesthesia for TJA based on current evidence.

What is new

A large retrospective cohort study of over 500,000 patients in South Korea (2016-2021) compared RA and GA in total hip or knee arthroplasty. Key findings:

- RA reduced 30-day and 90-day mortality by 31% and 22%, respectively, compared to GA.

- No significant difference in overall postoperative complications between groups.

- RA showed greater mortality benefits in total hip arthroplasty (THA) than in total knee arthroplasty (TKA).

- RA was linked to fewer cerebral infarctions and pulmonary embolisms but higher rates of acute coronary events and UTIs.

Clinical impact of anesthesia in TJA

1. Mortality outcomes

The data strongly indicate that regional anesthesia (RA) provides significant survival advantages over general anesthesia (GA) in the early postoperative period following TJA. The study demonstrated that patients who received RA had:

- 31% lower 30-day mortality (0.3% for RA vs. 0.5% for GA).

- 22% lower 90-day mortality (1.1% for RA vs. 1.4% for GA).

This reduced mortality can be attributed to several factors unique to RA. Unlike GA, RA avoids using endotracheal intubation and mechanical ventilation, which lowers the risk of respiratory complications such as pneumonia, a common postoperative concern. Additionally, RA minimizes the cardiovascular stress associated with GA, particularly in elderly or frail patients who are more susceptible to hemodynamic fluctuations and myocardial stress during and after surgery. Furthermore, RA's impact on improved hemodynamic stability likely plays a role in preventing fatal complications like myocardial infarctions or strokes, which are more commonly observed with GA.

2. Postoperative complications

Despite RA's clear benefits in reducing early postoperative mortality, the study found no significant difference in the overall complication rate between RA and GA (18.1% for RA vs. 17.8% for GA). However, certain specific complications showed notable variations:

- RA reduced the risk of cerebral infarction (stroke), pulmonary embolism, and heart failure. The reduced stroke and pulmonary embolism risks are likely due to better hemodynamic control and reduced need for anticoagulants post-surgery, which are more often required after GA due to prolonged immobility and increased risk of thromboembolism.

- Increased risk of acute coronary events was observed with RA. This could be linked to the hemodynamic effects of spinal or epidural anesthesia, which can cause hypotension and reflex tachycardia, potentially stressing the heart.

- Urinary tract infections (UTIs) were more common in the RA group. This is a well-known risk associated with RA, particularly spinal anesthesia, as it can cause temporary urinary retention. Postoperative retention often necessitates catheterization, which in turn increases the risk of UTIs.

These findings highlight the complexity of choosing the right anesthesia technique. While RA offers survival benefits and reduces some severe complications, it is not without risks, particularly for cardiovascular events and UTIs. Clinicians need to assess these risks on a case-by-case basis, balancing the overall benefits of RA against specific patient vulnerabilities.

3. Subgroup analysis: THA vs. TKA

A key insight from the study is that the benefits of RA over GA were more pronounced in patients undergoing total hip arthroplasty (THA) compared to total knee arthroplasty (TKA). In THA:

- 30-day mortality was 27% lower in the RA group compared to the GA group.

- 90-day mortality was 21% lower for RA compared to GA.

By contrast, in TKA:

- 30-day mortality was reduced by 26% with RA, but there was no significant difference in 90-day mortality or overall complication rates between RA and GA.

THA patients tend to be older, with more comorbidities, and the surgery itself is more complex and carries a higher risk of complications compared to TKA. RA's ability to reduce the risks of severe complications, such as thromboembolism and stroke, makes it particularly beneficial in this higher-risk population. On the other hand, TKA patients generally have fewer comorbidities and may not benefit as dramatically from RA's protective effects.

4. Implications for practice

The findings from this large-scale study underscore the need for individualized anesthesia selection in TJA. Given its clear survival advantages, RA should be strongly considered for patients undergoing THA, especially those with higher mortality risk. However, the choice of anesthesia should consider the patient's overall health, surgical complexity, and specific risk factors for complications.

When to favor RA:

- Older patients or those with significant comorbidities (e.g., cardiac disease or respiratory problems) who are at higher risk for postoperative mortality.

- THA patients, where the benefits of RA in reducing mortality are most evident.

- Patients at increased risk of thromboembolic events or stroke, as RA provides better hemodynamic control and reduces these risks.

Considerations for GA:

- Patients with pre-existing cardiovascular disease that the hypotensive effects of RA could exacerbate.

- Individuals at higher risk of UTIs or urinary retention, particularly if spinal anesthesia is planned.

- In cases where RA may not be feasible or appropriate, such as in patients with spinal abnormalities or infections at the injection site.

Limitations

- This study provides compelling evidence favoring RA in TJA, but it is not without limitations. Several factors that can influence postoperative outcomes, such as body mass index (BMI), smoking status, duration of surgery, and intraoperative blood loss, were not included in the analysis. Furthermore, the study focused exclusively on South Korean patients, which may limit its generalizability to other populations with different healthcare systems and patient demographics.

Key takeaways

- ☑ RA is associated with lower 30-day and 90-day mortality in total joint arthroplasty, particularly in total hip arthroplasty (THA).

- ☑ No significant difference in overall postoperative complication rates was found between RA and GA, although specific complications like stroke and pulmonary embolism were reduced with RA.

- ☑ Increased risks of acute coronary events and urinary tract infections were observed in patients receiving RA, indicating the need for careful patient selection.

- ☑ Subgroup analysis shows that RA's mortality benefits are more pronounced in THA compared to TKA, suggesting that RA may be the preferred option for hip replacement surgeries.

- ☑ Individualized decision-making is critical, balancing the benefits of RA against the risks, particularly in patients with pre-existing cardiovascular conditions or a predisposition to UTIs.

Additional recommended reading

1. Oh TK, Song IA. Regional versus general anesthesia for total hip and knee arthroplasty: a nationwide retrospective cohort study. *Reg Anesth Pain Med.* Published online April 30, 2024.

2. Memtsoudis SG, Sun X, Chiu YL, et al. Perioperative comparative effectiveness of anesthetic technique in orthopedic patients [published correction appears in *Anesthesiology.* 2016 Sep;125(3):610.

3. Lee J, Lee JS, Park SH, Shin SA, Kim K. Cohort Profile: The National Health Insurance Service-National Sample Cohort (NHIS-NSC), South Korea. *Int J Epidemiol.* 2017;46(2):e15.

PENG block vs. lateral QLB and opioid consumption after total hip arthroplasty

24

Why this topic is important

Total hip arthroplasty (THA) is one of the most common orthopedic procedures performed globally, particularly as populations age and rates of osteoarthritis and joint disease rise. By 2040, the demand for THA is projected to grow by 176%, and by 2060, it could increase by as much as 659%. The shift toward outpatient or rapid-recovery protocols following THA has placed even greater importance on effective pain management strategies that facilitate early mobility, minimize opioid consumption, and shorten hospital stays.

While opioids have traditionally been the mainstay for managing postoperative pain, their use carries significant risks, including respiratory depression, sedation, nausea, vomiting, and the potential for long-term addiction. As such, the growing emphasis on opioid-sparing techniques has led to the increased use of regional anesthesia. Nerve blocks offer significant benefits, such as reducing opioid requirements, providing targeted analgesia, and sparing motor function-all crucial for enhancing recovery and reducing opioid-related complications.

Two of the most effective blocks for THA include the lateral quadratus lumborum block (QLB) and the more recently introduced pericapsular nerve group (PENG) block. Both target sensory innervation to the hip, providing pain relief while allowing early ambulation. However, a head-to-head comparison of their efficacy in reducing opioid consumption and pain management has been lacking. A recent study by Hay et al.[1] provides critical insights into how these blocks compare and their role in modern multimodal analgesia protocols.

Objectives of this update

- To evaluate the comparative efficacy of PENG + lateral femoral cutaneous (LFC) block and lateral QLB in minimizing cumulative opioid consumption in the first 72 hours following THA.

- To understand the effects of these blocks on postoperative pain during rest and movement, patient mobility, and functional recovery.

- To offer clinical guidance on selecting the appropriate regional anesthesia technique for THA, focusing on optimizing patient outcomes and promoting opioid-sparing strategies.

- To explore the implications of these findings for same-day discharge and reduced hospital length of stay (LOS) in patients undergoing THA.

What is new

A 2024 randomized controlled trial[1] contributes new data comparing the PENG block (combined with the LFC block) to the lateral QLB in THA patients. Its findings have important implications for postoperative pain management, opioid consumption, and recovery protocols.

- Lower opioid consumption with QLB: The lateral QLB resulted in significantly lower cumulative opioid consumption compared to the PENG + LFC block from 36 to 72 hours post-surgery, highlighting its opioid-sparing benefits during the critical postoperative period.

- Better pain control during movement with QLB: The study found that patients who received a lateral QLB experienced lower pain scores during movement, which is essential for early ambulation and functional recovery.

- Similar pain at rest and functional outcomes: Both blocks were equally effective in controlling pain at rest, and there were no significant differences in patient-reported functional outcomes (HOOS JR and PROMIS-10 scores).

- Comparable early ambulation and discharge rates: Both blocks facilitated early mobilization and similar rates of same-day discharge, making them viable options in modern outpatient recovery protocols.

Study design and methodology

The study by Hay et al.[1] was a randomized controlled trial involving 106 patients undergoing elective primary THA. Participants were assigned to receive either a lateral QLB or a PENG block combined with an LFC nerve block. Both block techniques were administered preoperatively, and perioperative pain management protocols, including multimodal analgesia, were standardized across all patients.

Interventions

- Lateral Quadratus Lumborum Block (QLB) (fig-1): This block targets the lateral aspect of the quadratus lumborum muscle and provides analgesia by blocking somatic and visceral pain pathways. Ropivacaine (30 mL of 0.25%) was used to perform the block.

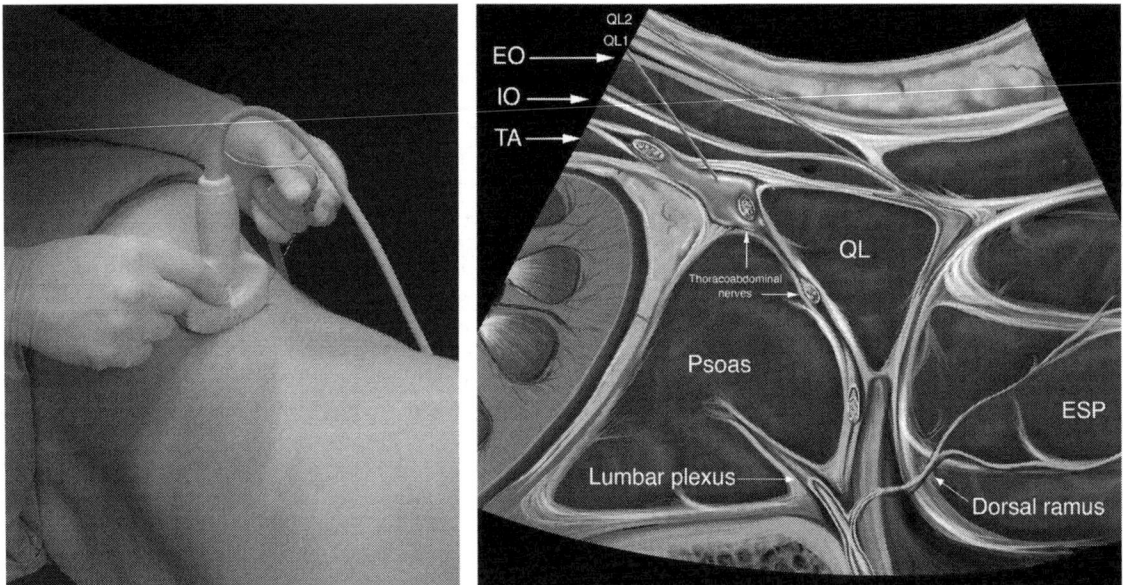

Fig-1. Initial transducer position and reverse ultrasound anatomy for a lateral (also known as a QL1). EO, internal oblique; IO, internal oblique; TA, transversus abdominis; QL, quadratus lumborum muscles.
Image taken from NYSORA LMS. https://nysoralms.com/

- Pericapsular Nerve Group (PENG) Block (fig-2) + LFC Block (fig-3): The PENG block targets the articular branches of the femoral, obturator, and accessory obturator nerves, providing sensory blockade to the anterior hip capsule without affecting motor function. This study combined it with an LFC block to provide additional analgesia for the lateral thigh. Ropivacaine (20 mL of 0.25% for PENG and 10 mL of 0.25% for LFC) was used.

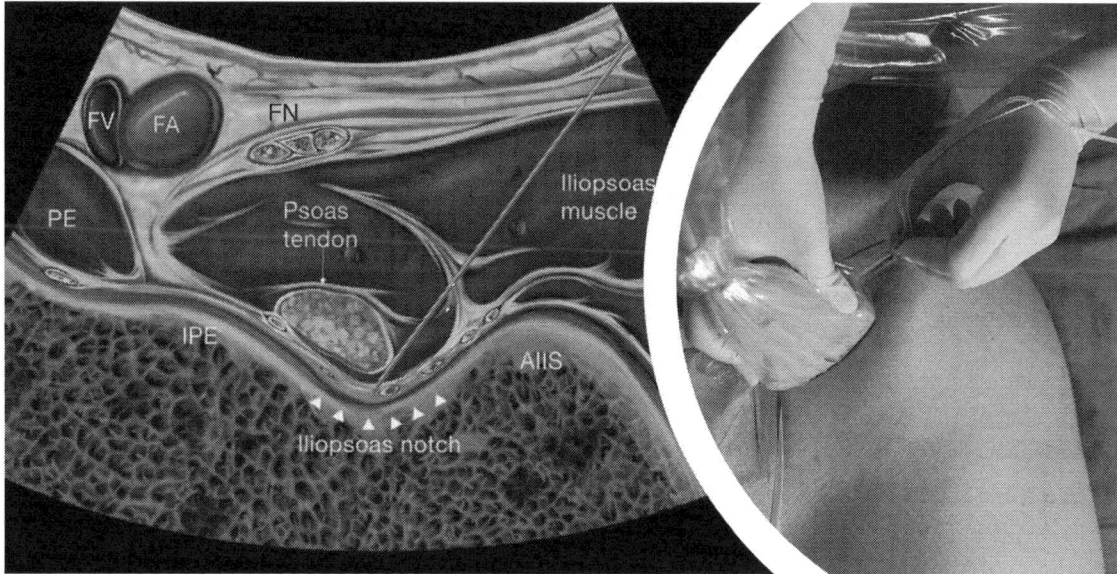

Fig-2. PENG block, reverse ultrasound anatomy. FA, femoral artery; FV, femoral vein; FN, femoral nerve; PE, pectineus muscle; IPE, iliopubic eminence; AIIS, anterior inferior iliac spine. Image taken from NYSORA LMS. https://nysoralms.com/

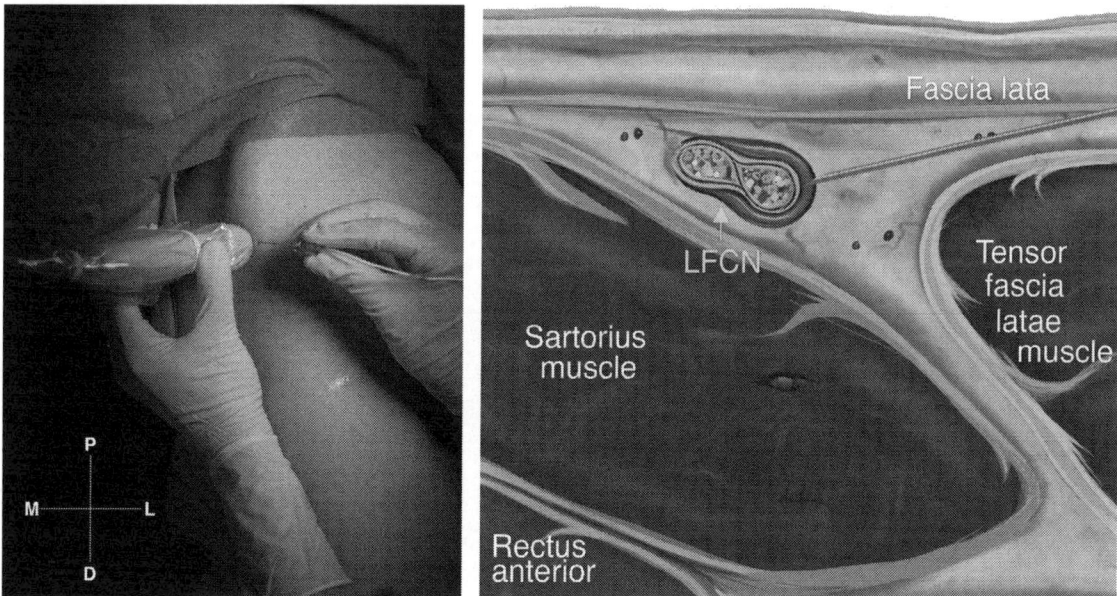

Fig-3. Reverse ultrasound anatomy for a lateral femoral cutaneous nerve (LFCN) block.
Image taken from NYSORA LMS. https://nysoralms.com/

Outcomes

- Primary outcome: Cumulative opioid consumption, measured in intravenous morphine milligram equivalents (IV MME), over the first 72 hours postoperatively.

- Secondary outcomes: These included postoperative pain scores (both at rest and during movement), time to first ambulation, hospital length of stay (LOS), same-day discharge rates, functional outcomes (measured using HOOS JR and PROMIS-10 surveys), and opioid-related side effects (nausea, vomiting, itching, respiratory depression).

Key comparative outcomes between lateral QLB and PENG + LFC block.

Parameter	Lateral QLB	PENG + LFC block
Cumulative opioid consumption (36-72 hrs)	Lower opioid consumption (33 MME less at 72 hrs)	Higher opioid consumption
Pain with movement (VAS)	Lower pain with movement (7 mm lower at 72 hrs)	Higher pain with movement
Pain at rest (VAS)	Similar to PENG	Similar to QLB
Time to first ambulation (minutes)	~456 minutes	~465 minutes
Length of stay (LOS)	Comparable	Comparable
Same-day discharge rate	~50%	~50%
Functional outcome measures	Similar (HOOS JR, PROMIS-10)	Similar (HOOS JR, PROMIS-10)
Opioid-related side effects	Comparable	Comparable

Opioid consumption

The lateral QLB was associated with significantly lower cumulative opioid consumption compared to the PENG + LFC block. This difference was particularly notable from 36 to 72 hours postoperatively:

- 36 hours: Mean difference of 18.0 MME.

- 48 hours: Mean difference of 23.0 MME.

- 60 hours: Mean difference of 28.0 MME.

- 72 hours: Mean difference of 33.0 MME.

These results suggest that the lateral QLB offers superior opioid-sparing benefits compared to the PENG + LFC block, especially in the later postoperative period when block effects may begin to wane.

Pain scores

Pain with movement: Patients who received the lateral QLB reported significantly lower pain scores with movement than those who received the PENG + LFC block. This difference is critical for encouraging early mobility, a key factor in rapid recovery protocols.

- At 72 hours, the QLB group reported pain scores that were, on average, 7 mm lower on the Visual Analog Scale (VAS) compared to the PENG + LFC group (p = 0.032). While this difference is statistically significant, it is less clinically relevant, as a 7 mm difference on the VAS falls below the threshold typically considered meaningful for patient-reported pain relief.

Pain at rest: No significant differences were observed between the two groups in pain scores at rest throughout the postoperative period.

Time to ambulation and functional outcomes

Time to first ambulation: Both groups showed similar times to ambulation, with the lateral QLB group ambulating at a median of 456 minutes postoperatively, compared to 465 minutes for the PENG group (p = 0.185). These findings suggest that both blocks effectively preserve motor function and enable early mobilization.

Functional outcomes: The HOOS JR and PROMIS-10 surveys did not find significant differences in patient-reported functional outcomes between the two groups. This indicates that both blocks support a similar level of functional recovery at 1 week, 2 weeks, and 6 weeks postoperatively.

Hospital LOS and same-day discharge

- Length of stay (LOS): Both groups had comparable hospital stays, with no significant differences in LOS.

- Same-day discharge rates: The study found no significant differences in same-day discharge rates between the QLB and PENG + LFC groups, with approximately 50% of patients in each group being discharged on the same day of surgery.

Opioid-related side effects

Opioid-related side effects (such as nausea, vomiting, itching, and respiratory issues) did not differ significantly between the two groups. This underscores the importance of using regional anesthesia as part of a multimodal analgesia strategy to minimize opioid-related complications.

Clinical implications and discussion

This study[1] highlights the superior opioid-sparing benefits of the lateral QLB over the PENG + LFC block in patients undergoing THA. The significant reduction in opioid consumption from 36 to 72 hours postoperatively is a key finding, particularly as opioid use in the later postoperative period often correlates with rebound pain and discomfort following the resolution of regional blocks.

When to use lateral QLBs

- The lateral QLB should be strongly considered in patients where minimizing opioid use is a primary goal, especially in the setting of enhanced recovery pathways that prioritize early mobility and same-day discharge.

- Patients who experience higher levels of movement-related pain may particularly benefit from the lateral QLB, as this block demonstrated superior control of dynamic pain during ambulation and rehabilitation.

When to use PENG + LFC block

- The PENG + LFC block remains a viable option for pain management following THA, particularly in scenarios where ease of application and sensory coverage for anterior and lateral thigh pain is desired.

- While opioid consumption was higher with the PENG block, it still provides effective analgesia, and combining it with other elements of multimodal analgesia can help achieve adequate pain control.

Key takeaways

☑ Both lateral QLB and PENG + LFC blocks are effective options for pain management following THA, supporting modern outpatient recovery pathways.

☑ Opioid consumption: The lateral QLB demonstrated lower opioid consumption from 36 to 72 hours postoperatively compared to the PENG + LFC block, though both techniques contribute to an overall reduction in opioid use.

☑ Pain control: The QLB group reported lower pain scores with movement, but the 7 mm difference on the VAS, while statistically significant, is not clinically meaningful.

☑ No differences were observed in resting pain scores or functional outcomes between the two blocks, supporting the use of either block in rapid recovery protocols where motor function is preserved.

☑ Both blocks enable early ambulation and same-day discharge, making them suitable for outpatient THA procedures in modern recovery pathways.

☑ Multimodal analgesia remains crucial: Both blocks should be viewed as part of a broader analgesia strategy that includes systemic medications and periarticular injections to optimize postoperative pain control and minimize opioid use.

Additional recommended reading

1. Hay E, Kelly T, Wolf BJ, Hansen E, Brown A, Lautenschlager C, Wilson SH. Comparison of pericapsular nerve group and lateral quadratus lumborum blocks on cumulative opioid consumption after primary total hip arthroplasty: a randomized controlled trial. Reg Anesth Pain Med. 2024 Oct 10

2. Huda AU, Minhas R. Quadratus Lumborum Block Reduces Postoperative Pain Scores and Opioids Consumption in Total Hip Arthroplasty: A Meta-Analysis. *Cureus.* 2022;14(2):e22287.

3. Girón-Arango, L., Peng, P. W. H., Chin, K. J., et al. (2018). Pericapsular Nerve Group (PENG) Block for Hip Fracture. *Regional Anesthesia & Pain Medicine*, 43(8), 859-863.

Nerve blocks in the preoperative management of hip fractures

25

Why this topic is important

Hip fractures are common, particularly in older adults, and are associated with severe preoperative pain, functional decline, and increased mortality. Effective pain management is critical to reducing complications like delirium, impaired mobility, and longer hospital stays. While opioids are frequently used, they are associated with significant side effects, especially in older populations.

Peripheral nerve blocks (PNBs) have emerged as an effective alternative for preoperative pain relief in hip fracture patients. Techniques such as femoral nerve block (FNB) (fig-1A), fascia iliaca compartment block (FICB) (fig-1B), and pericapsular nerve group (PENG) block (fig-1C) target specific nerve pathways to alleviate pain. However, the comparative efficacy and safety of these blocks remain unclear.

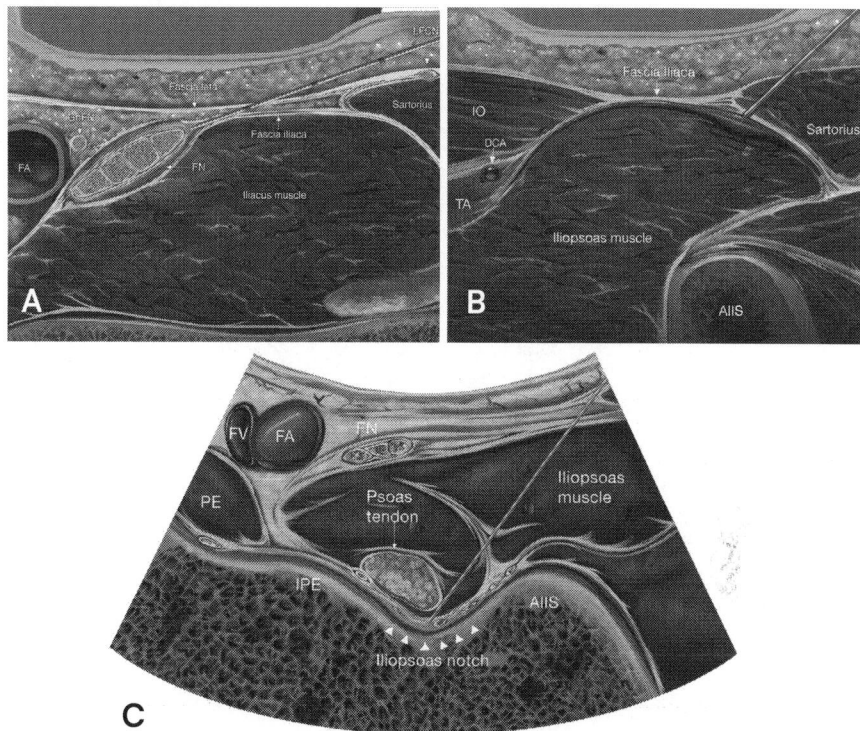

Fig-1. A) Reverse ultrasound anatomy for a femoral nerve block. FA, femoral artery; FN, femoral nerve; GnFN, genitofemoral nerve. B) Reverse ultrasound anatomy for a suprainguinal approach to a fascia iliaca block. IO, internal oblique; TA, transverse abdominis; AIIS, anterior inferior iliac spine; DCA, deep circumflex artery. C) Reverse ultrasound anatomy to a pericapsular nerve group (PENG) block. FA, femoral artery; FV, femoral vein; FN, femoral nerve; PE, pectineus muscle; IPE, iliopubic eminence; AIIS, anterior inferior iliac spine.
Images taken from NYSORA LMS. https://nysoralms.com/

A recent systematic review and network meta-analysis assessed the efficacy of these blocks for pain management before hip fracture surgery[1]. This update summarizes its findings, focusing on clinical implications and areas for future research.

Objectives of this update

- Evaluate the efficacy of different PNBs in reducing pain and opioid consumption preoperatively.

- Discuss the safety profile of these blocks, including potential adverse events.

- Provide recommendations for integrating PNBs into clinical practice.

What is new

This comprehensive meta-analysis reviewed 63 randomized controlled trials involving 4,778 participants. Key findings include:

- Pain reduction: PENG block significantly reduced pain scores compared to FICB, FNB, and no block at two hours post-block.

- Opioid consumption: PENG block was superior to other blocks in reducing opioid use, though the evidence was limited.

- Safety: PNBs were associated with few serious adverse events when performed under ultrasound guidance.

Detailed findings

Study design

This meta-analysis included trials comparing PNBs (FNB, FICB, 3-in-1 block, PENG block) to each other or no block. Outcomes included:

1. Pain scores at two hours post-block.

2. Preoperative opioid consumption.

3. Length of hospital stay.

4. Adverse events and patient satisfaction.

Primary outcomes

1. Pain scores:

   ◦ PENG block achieved the greatest reduction in pain scores at two hours.

   ◦ FICB and FNB were also effective but less so compared to PENG block.

2. Opioid consumption:

   ◦ PENG block reduced opioid use more effectively than FICB and FNB.

   ◦ No significant difference in morphine consumption was observed between FICB, FNB, and no block.

3. Length of stay:

   ◦ No significant difference in hospital stay was observed across groups.

Secondary outcomes

1. Safety:

   ◦ Adverse events such as vascular punctures were rare, particularly with ultrasound guidance.

   ◦ Quadriceps weakness was reported in FICB, highlighting its potential to impair mobility.

2. Patient satisfaction:

   ◦ PENG block yielded higher satisfaction scores compared to FICB and no block.

Implications for practice

Clinical recommendations

1. Block selection:

   ◦ PENG block should be prioritized for its superior analgesic efficacy and opioid-sparing benefits.

   ◦ FICB and FNB remain viable options when PENG block expertise or resources are unavailable.

2. Ultrasound guidance:

   ◦ Ultrasound should be used to enhance safety and ensure accurate nerve targeting.

3. Integration into emergency departments:

   ◦ PNBs can be administered in emergency settings to manage pain early, improving patient comfort and reducing opioid exposure.

Patient selection

- Older adults: PNBs are particularly beneficial for minimizing opioid-related side effects in geriatric populations.

- Patients with high fall risk: Consider PENG or FNB to avoid quadriceps weakness, as seen with FICB.

Challenges and limitations

1. Heterogeneity of studies:

   ◦ Variability in block techniques, local anesthetic concentrations, and outcome measurement methods may influence results.

2. Risk of bias:

   ◦ Many included studies had a high risk of bias, particularly due to non-blinded outcome assessments.

3. Limited data on long-term outcomes:

   ◦ The impact of PNBs on functional recovery and chronic pain management requires further exploration.

Key takeaways

☑ PENG block is the most effective peripheral nerve block for preoperative pain relief in hip fracture patients.

☑ FICB and FNB remain viable alternatives with fewer complications than systemic opioids.

☑ Ultrasound guidance improves the safety and efficacy of PNBs, reducing adverse events like vascular punctures.

☑ Incorporating PNBs into early pain management protocols enhances patient satisfaction and minimizes opioid consumption.

Additional recommended reading

1. Hayashi M, Yamamoto N, Kuroda N, et al. Peripheral nerve blocks in the preoperative management of hip fractures: A systematic review and network meta-analysis. *Ann Emerg Med.* 2024;83:522-538.

2. Exsteen OW, Svendsen CN, Rothe C, et al. Ultrasound-guided peripheral nerve blocks for preoperative pain management in hip fractures: A systematic review. *BMC Anesthesiol.* 2022;22:192.

3. Griffiths R, Babu S, Dixon P, et al. Guideline for the management of hip fractures 2020 guideline by the Association of Anaesthetists. *Anaesthesia.* 2021;76:225-237.

Autologous breast reconstruction: Paravertebral and ESPB or local infiltration

26

Why this topic is important

Autologous breast reconstruction (ABR), particularly after mastectomy, is a complex surgical procedure that is associated with significant postoperative pain. The latissimus dorsi myocutaneous flap, a commonly used reconstruction technique, involves the dissection and transfer of a large muscle group, which compounds the pain from mastectomy alone. Managing this pain effectively is crucial to enhance recovery and shorten hospital stays, allowing patients to return home sooner, with less opioid dependence and fewer complications.

Historically, pain control in these procedures has relied heavily on opioids and local infiltration analgesia (LIA), where the surgeon administers local anesthetics directly into the wound. While effective to some extent, this approach has several drawbacks, including higher opioid use, prolonged hospitalization, and the risk of opioid-related side effects such as nausea, vomiting, and constipation.

In recent years, regional anesthesia techniques like the paravertebral block (PVB) and erector spinae plane block (ESPB) have emerged as alternatives to LIA. These blocks are part of multimodal analgesia protocols that aim to reduce opioid use and enhance patient recovery. Understanding the effectiveness of PVB and ESP compared to traditional LIA is critical for optimizing postoperative care in breast reconstruction patients.

Objectives of this update

- Introduce the role of regional anesthesia blocks (PVB and ESPB) in autologous breast reconstruction.

- Compare the clinical outcomes of PVB and ESP blocks with traditional local infiltration techniques.

- Highlight the potential for reduced opioid use, shorter hospital stays, and enhanced recovery in patients receiving regional blocks.

- Discuss the safety, technical considerations, and clinical applications of ESP as a potentially safer alternative to PVB.

What is new

The latest research has provided new insights into the comparative effectiveness of regional anesthesia techniques versus traditional local infiltration analgesia. A retrospective cohort study[1] conducted between 2018 and 2022 has revealed that using PVB and ESP blocks in autologous breast reconstruction significantly decreases the length of hospital stay (LOS) and reduces intraoperative opioid consumption.

Understanding PVB and ESP blocks

Paravertebral block (PVB)

The paravertebral block has long been regarded as the gold standard for regional anesthesia in breast surgeries. It involves injecting local anesthetics into the paravertebral space (fig-1A), targeting both the dorsal and ventral rami of the spinal nerves, as well as the sympathetic chain. This block provides extensive coverage, numbing the anterior chest wall and the breast, which is essential in surgeries like mastectomy and breast reconstruction.

However, despite its effectiveness, PVB is technically challenging. The proximity of the pleura means that there is a risk of pneumothorax (collapsed lung), and the injection can inadvertently spread into the epidural or intrathecal spaces, leading to more serious complications like spinal anesthesia or hypotension. Therefore, PVB requires a high level of skill and experience, typically limiting its use to advanced practitioners.

Despite these challenges, PVB continues to be a powerful tool in reducing opioid use and enhancing recovery in breast surgery patients. The study confirmed its ability to reduce hospital stays and improve overall patient outcomes compared to traditional LIA.

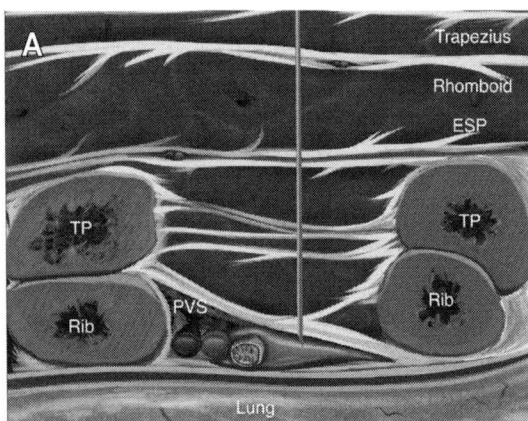

Erector spinae plane block (ESPB)

The erector spinae plane block is a newer and increasingly popular technique. It involves injecting local anesthetic deep to the erector spinae muscle and above the transverse processes of the vertebrae (fig-1B). This block targets the dorsal rami of the spinal nerves and offers substantial analgesia for the posterior chest wall and donor site pain, making it particularly useful in latissimus dorsi flap reconstructions.

One of the key advantages of the ESP block is its simplicity. The landmarks for the block are easier to identify, and the injection is more superficial than in PVB, reducing the risk of complications. Because of these features, ESP is often considered a safer alternative, especially in settings where expertise in advanced regional anesthesia may be limited.

While the ESP block may not provide as extensive coverage of the anterior chest wall as PVB, the study suggests that it still offers substantial reductions in LOS and opioid use, making it a viable option for many patients. ESP's safety and ease of application make it particularly appealing for ambulatory or outpatient breast surgeries.

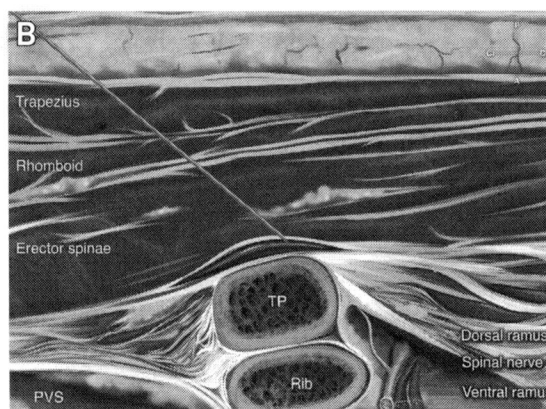

Fig-1A. Paravertebral block, reverse ultrasound anatomy. Using an out-of-plane needle approach, local anesthetic spread around the spinal nerves as they arise from the intervertebral foramen. TP, transverse process; PVS, paravertebral space; ESP, erector spinae muscles. Fig-1B. Erector spinae plane block, reverse ultrasound anatomy. Local anesthetic spread in the plane deep to the erector spinae muscles and superficial to the transverse processes. TP, transverse process; PVS, paravertebral space. Images taken from NYSORA LMS. https://nysoralms.com/

Autologous breast reconstruction: Paravertebral and ESPB or local infiltration

Study overview

A study by Ayyala et al.[1] retrospectively analyzed 122 patients who underwent autologous breast reconstruction using the latissimus dorsi flap. These patients were divided into three groups based on the analgesic method used: local infiltration (72 patients), PVB (26 patients), and ESP (24 patients).

Key outcomes:

- Length of stay: The median LOS for patients who received local infiltration was 48 hours. For those who had PVB or ESP blocks, the LOS was reduced to 26 hours. This dramatic reduction underscores the effectiveness of regional anesthesia in promoting faster recovery and enabling earlier discharge.

- Opioid use: Intraoperative opioid consumption was significantly lower in the PVB and ESP groups. Patients who received local infiltration required an average of 52 MME intraoperatively, while those with PVB or ESP required only 30 and 40 MME, respectively.

- Postoperative pain: The study also assessed postoperative pain scores, finding that both PVB and ESP blocks contributed to better pain control than local infiltration. While patients with ESP blocks had slightly higher maximum pain scores than those with PVB, both groups experienced meaningful reductions in pain compared to the local infiltration group.

- Safety: Neither PVB nor ESP was associated with serious complications. The ESP block, in particular, had a favorable safety profile due to its more superficial approach.

Comparative overview of analgesia techniques in autologous breast reconstruction

Parameter	Paravertebral block	Erector spinae plane block	Local infiltration
Technical difficulty	High (Requires advanced skills)	Low (easier to perform)	Low (surgeon administered)
Coverage area	Ventral + dorsal rami, sympathetic ganglia	Dorsal rami, posterior site	Local site only
Risk of complications	Pneumothorax, epidural spread	Minimal (superficial technique)	Minimal
Opioid reduction (MME)	-23 MME	-23 MME	None
Length of stay (reduction)	-20 hours	-24 hours	Baseline
Pain control (effectiveness)	Excellent (anterior and posterior)	Good (posterior)	Moderate
Ideal for	Major breast surgeries with anterior pain	Surgeries with posterior site pain	Low-risk patients needing basic analgesia

Implications for clinical practice

The findings from this study have important implications for the perioperative management of patients undergoing autologous breast reconstruction.

1. Shortened length of stay: By incorporating PVB or ESP blocks into multimodal analgesia protocols, healthcare providers can significantly reduce the length of hospitalization. This reduction is not only beneficial for patient comfort and satisfaction but also has economic advantages, potentially lowering the cost of care.

2. Reduced opioid use: The opioid-sparing effects of these blocks are particularly important in the context of the ongoing opioid crisis. Reducing opioid consumption minimizes the risk of opioid-related side effects, dependence, and longer-term complications such as chronic pain.

3. ESP as a safer alternative: Given its ease of administration and lower risk of complications, the ESP block is an attractive option for many patients. It offers comparable reductions in LOS and opioid use to PVB, with fewer technical challenges. This makes it especially useful in outpatient or ambulatory surgery settings, where simpler and safer techniques are preferred.

4. Tailoring pain management: The choice between PVB and ESP may depend on the patient's specific needs and the procedure's complexity. For more extensive surgeries involving the anterior chest wall, PVB may still be preferred. However, ESP offers a compelling alternative with a favorable safety profile for latissimus dorsi flap reconstructions, where posterior donor site pain is the primary concern.

Key takeaways

☑ Shortened hospital stay: Compared to local infiltration, both PVB and ESP blocks reduce the postoperative length of stay by approximately 20-24 hours.

☑ Opioid-sparing effect: Intraoperative opioid consumption is significantly lower in patients receiving PVB or ESP, reducing opioid-related side effects and promoting faster recovery.

☑ Effective pain control: Both blocks provide superior pain relief to local infiltration, though PVB may offer better coverage for anterior chest wall pain.

☑ ESP is a safer, simpler alternative: ESP block is easier to perform and carries fewer risks than PVB, making it suitable for outpatient surgeries and centers with less access to advanced regional anesthesia expertise.

☑ Clinical flexibility: The choice between PVB and ESP should be tailored to the patient's needs and the specifics of the surgical procedure, with ESP offering a safe and effective option for many cases.

Additional recommended reading

1. Ayyala HS, Assel M, Aloise J, et al. Paravertebral and erector spinae plane blocks decrease length of stay compared with local infiltration analgesia in autologous breast reconstruction. *Reg Anesth Pain Med* 2024.

2. Schnabel A, Reichl SU, Kranke P, et al. Efficacy and safety of paravertebral blocks in breast surgery: a meta-analysis of randomized controlled trials. *Br J Anaesth*. 2010.

3. Glissmeyer C, Johnson W, Sherman B, et al. Effect of paravertebral nerve blocks on narcotic use after mastectomy with reconstruction. *Am J Surg*. 2015.

Anterior quadratus lumborum block for analgesia after living-donor renal transplantation

27

Why this topic is important

Living-donor renal transplantation remains the definitive treatment for end-stage renal disease, offering superior outcomes compared to dialysis. Despite its benefits, significant postoperative pain is common, challenging clinicians to provide effective and safe analgesia. Traditional methods, such as opioids, are fraught with risks, including respiratory depression, nausea, and potential impacts on graft function. Non-opioid alternatives, like nonsteroidal anti-inflammatory drugs (NSAIDs), are also limited in this population due to nephrotoxicity concerns.

Thoracic epidural analgesia has historically been considered the gold standard for abdominal surgeries. Still, it is less suitable for renal transplantation patients due to bleeding risks associated with heparin use and platelet dysfunction. Consequently, there is growing interest in regional anesthesia techniques, such as abdominal wall blocks, which provide localized analgesia with minimal systemic effects. Among these, the anterior quadratus lumborum (QL) block has gained attention for its potential to deliver both somatic and visceral pain relief via injectate spread to the thoracic paravertebral space (fig-1). However, the efficacy of this approach in renal transplant patients remains underexplored.

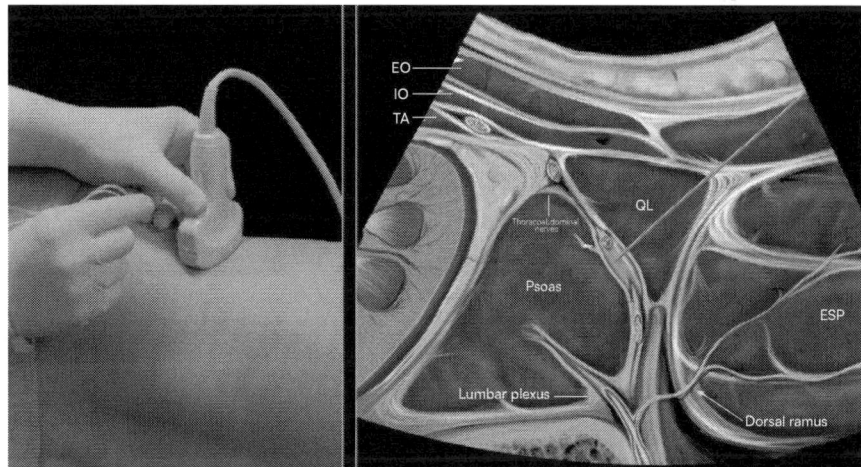

Fig-1. Reverse ultrasound anatomy with needle insertion in-plane for a an anterior quadratus lumborum block. Ideal local anesthetic distribution (blue) on the anterior aspect of the QL muscle. EO, external oblique; IO, internal oblique; TA, transversus abdominis; QL, quadratus lumborum; ESP, erector spinae muscles. Image taken from NYSORA LMS. https://nysoralms.com/

This update reviews the findings of a recent randomized controlled trial evaluating the anterior QL block's efficacy in reducing opioid consumption and improving postoperative recovery after living-donor renal transplantation[1].

Objectives of this update

- Understand the role of the anterior QL block in managing postoperative pain for renal transplant patients.

- Evaluate the findings of recent clinical research on its impact on opioid consumption, pain scores, and recovery metrics.

- Discuss clinical applicability and identify patient-specific contexts where the anterior QL block may or may not provide value.

What is new

The study[1], a double-blinded randomized controlled trial, is the first to assess the effectiveness of the anterior QL block in renal transplant recipients. Key features include:

- Comparison of 88 patients undergoing living-donor renal transplantation, randomized to receive either an anterior QL block with 30 mL of ropivacaine 0.375% or a placebo block with saline.

- A focus on opioid consumption within 24 hours postoperatively as the primary outcome, alongside secondary metrics such as pain scores, quality of recovery, and length of stay.

- Multimodal analgesia, including acetaminophen and intravenous patient-controlled fentanyl, was administered to all patients.

Detailed findings

Study design

Participants underwent ultrasound-guided anterior QL block or sham block postoperatively. Pain and recovery were assessed using standardized tools, including cumulative opioid consumption measured in morphine milligram equivalents (MME), quality of recovery (QoR-15), and patient satisfaction scores.

Primary outcome: Opioid consumption

- No significant difference was observed in 24-hour opioid use between the QL block and control groups (median 160.5 MME vs. 187.5 MME).

- Similarly, opioid consumption over 48 hours showed no significant intergroup differences.

Secondary outcomes

1. Pain scores:
   - Numerical rating scale (NRS) scores at rest and during movement were comparable between groups at all time points up to 48 hours postoperatively.

2. Quality of Recovery (QoR-15):
   - Scores measured 24 hours after surgery showed no difference between groups, suggesting the QL block did not enhance recovery perception.

3. Time to first ambulation and length of stay:
   - No significant differences were noted between groups for these metrics, with median hospital stays of 10 days in both cohorts.

4. Sensory blockade and motor weakness:
   - The QL block effectively induced sensory blockade in 83 of 88 patients.
   - One case of transient motor weakness was reported in the QL block group, resolving without intervention.

5. Adverse effects:
   - Postoperative nausea and vomiting (PONV) rates were similar across groups, reflecting effective antiemetic prophylaxis in both cohorts.

Implications for practice

The anterior QL block, despite theoretical advantages, did not demonstrate significant benefits in opioid reduction or recovery enhancement in the context of a robust multimodal analgesic protocol. This raises important considerations for its role in clinical practice:

1. Multimodal analgesia as a foundation:

   ○ The lack of additional analgesic benefits from the QL block may reflect the efficacy of multimodal analgesia, which provided adequate pain control in most patients.

2. Surgical context and pain characteristics:

   ○ Pain in renal transplantation is complex, involving visceral and somatic components. The QL block's limitations in influencing visceral pain may explain the lack of significant outcomes.

3. Utility in specific populations:

   ○ While the QL block may not be universally applicable, it could serve as an adjunct for patients at high risk of opioid-related side effects or in settings with limited multimodal options.

Challenges and limitations

Anatomical considerations:

- Injectate spread in the QL block can vary based on tissue compliance and block level. Insufficient cephalad spread may result in incomplete dermatomal coverage, particularly for incisions at the T10-L2 levels.

Study design constraints:

- The trial's single-center design and exclusion of deceased-donor transplants limit generalizability.

- Pain characterization (somatic vs. visceral) was not separately assessed, which could have clarified the block's limitations.

Broader evidence base:

- Inconsistent findings across studies on abdominal wall blocks for renal transplantation highlight the need for further research to optimize techniques and indications.

Key takeaways

- ☑ The anterior QL block did not significantly reduce opioid consumption or improve recovery outcomes in renal transplant recipients receiving multimodal analgesia.

- ☑ Multimodal analgesia remains the cornerstone of postoperative pain management in this population.

- ☑ The QL block may have situational utility but is not recommended for routine use in renal transplantation.

Additional recommended reading

1. Kim Y, Kim JT, Yang SM, et al. Anterior quadratus lumborum block for analgesia after living-donor renal transplantation: A double-blinded randomized controlled trial. *Reg Anesth Pain Med.* 2024;49:550-557.

2. Elsharkawy H, El-Boghdadly K, Barrington M. Quadratus lumborum block: Anatomical concepts, mechanisms, and techniques. *Anesthesiology.* 2019;130:322-35.

3. Korgvee A, Junttila E, Koskinen H, et al. Ultrasound-guided quadratus lumborum block for postoperative analgesia: A systematic review and meta-analysis. *Eur J Anaesthesiol.* 2021;38:115-29.

Programmed intermittent bolus or continuous infusion for ESPB in thoracoscopic surgery

28

Why this topic is important

Video-assisted thoracoscopic surgery (VATS) is a minimally invasive approach associated with less postoperative pain and faster recovery than open thoracotomy. Despite its advantages, significant postoperative pain remains a challenge for many patients. The erector spinae plane (ESP) block (fig-1), a regional analgesia technique, has gained popularity for its ability to mitigate this pain. However, an ongoing debate exists about the optimal method of delivering local anesthetic through ESP block catheters-either as a continuous infusion (CI) or programmed intermittent bolus (PIB). While PIB has shown promise in enhancing analgesic efficacy in some regional techniques, its impact on overall recovery and outcomes compared to CI remains unclear. A recent trial by Eochagain et al. (2024) evaluates the comparative effectiveness of these delivery methods in improving the quality of recovery (QoR) and other perioperative outcomes in patients undergoing VATS.

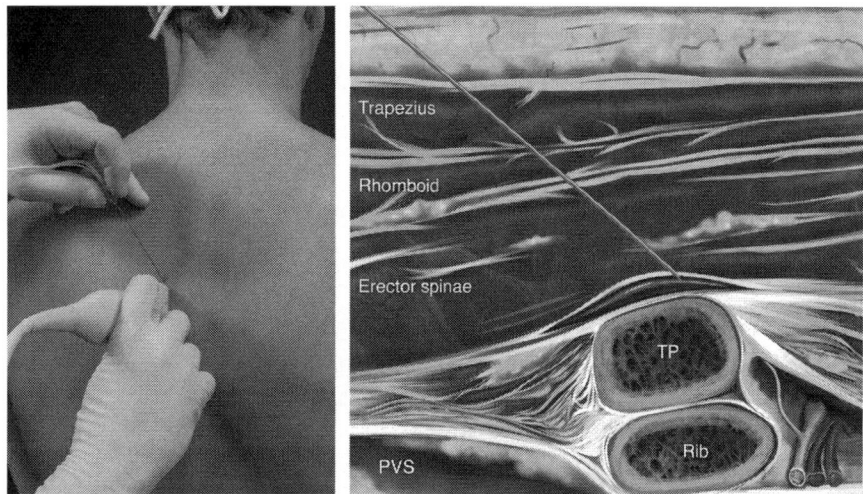

Fig-1. Reverse ultrasound anatomy of an ESPB with needle insertion in-plane from a cranial to caudad direction. The spinal nerve exits the paravertebral space with the dorsal ramus branching and traveling posterior to innervate the posterior back muscles. TP, transverse process; PVS, paravertebral space. Image taken from NYSORA LMS. https://nysoralms.com/

Objectives of this update

- Assess the impact of PIB versus CI on Quality of Recovery-15 (QoR-15) scores at 24 hours post-VATS.

- Compare secondary outcomes, including opioid consumption, pain levels, postoperative respiratory function, and antiemetic requirements.

- Provide clinical recommendations for selecting the optimal local anesthetic delivery method for ESP blocks in thoracoscopic surgery.

What is new

This study presents novel findings, including:

- No significant difference in 24-hour QoR-15 scores between PIB and CI groups, suggesting that delivery mode may not critically impact recovery.

- Lower rates of nausea and rescue antiemetic use in the PIB group, highlighting a potential advantage in managing postoperative nausea and vomiting (PONV).

- Comparable secondary outcomes, such as pain scores, opioid consumption, and time to mobilization, between the two methods.

Trial design and methodology

- Design and participants:
  - Single-center, double-blinded, randomized controlled trial involving 60 patients undergoing VATS.
  - Participants received ultrasound-guided ESP block catheters and were randomly assigned to PIB or CI regimens.

- Intervention protocols:
  - PIB group: Received levobupivacaine 0.125% (20 mL) every 2 hours via a pump delivering boluses.
  - CI group: Received levobupivacaine 0.125% at a continuous rate of 10 mL/hour.

- Outcome measures:
  - Primary outcome: QoR-15 score at 24 hours postoperatively.
  - Secondary outcomes: Pain scores, opioid consumption, respiratory function, antiemetic requirements, and length of hospital stay.

Results

- Quality of recovery:
  - Median QoR-15 scores: No significant difference between PBI and CI.
  - Improvements in individual QoR-15 domains were similar across both groups except for the nausea/vomiting domain, which favored PIB.

- Pain and opioid consumption:
  - Verbal rating scale (VRS) pain scores at rest and during deep inspiration were comparable between groups.
  - Total morphine milligram equivalents (MME) consumed postoperatively: No significant difference between groups.

- Postoperative nausea and vomiting (PONV):
  - 14% of PIB patients required rescue antiemetics, compared to 41% in the CI group.

- Respiratory and mobilization outcomes:
  - Inspiratory volume recovery at 24 hours was similar between PIB and CI groups.
  - Time to first mobilization was slightly shorter in the PIB group (13.3 hours vs 15.8 hours), though not statistically significant.

Clinical implications

- Efficacy of PIB and CI:
  - Both delivery methods provide effective analgesia for VATS patients, with no clinically meaningful differences in the overall quality of recovery.

- PONV management:
  - The reduced incidence of nausea and antiemetic use in the PIB group may influence its selection in patients at high risk for PONV.

- Practical considerations:
  - Selection between PIB and CI can be guided by institutional preferences, resource availability, and patient-specific factors rather than outcome differences.
- Volume and dosing consistency:
  - The comparable results underscore the importance of total anesthetic volume and dose over delivery method.

Limitations

- Short follow-up period: Outcomes were assessed only at 24 hours postoperatively, limiting insights into long-term recovery and complications.
- Single-center design: Results may not be generalizable to other institutions with differing patient populations and practices.
- Catheter-related challenges: The study observed catheter dislodgement and leakage in some cases, potentially affecting analgesia quality.

Key takeaways

☑ PIB and CI methods provide equivalent analgesic efficacy and quality of recovery for VATS patients.

☑ Reduced nausea and antiemetic use with PIB may offer an advantage in certain patient populations.

☑ Total anesthetic volume and dose may be more critical than the delivery method in determining outcomes.

☑ Selection of PIB or CI should be based on logistical and patient-specific factors, as clinical outcomes are comparable.

Additional recommended reading

1. Ni Eochagain A, Moorthy A, Shaker J, et al. Programmed intermittent bolus versus continuous infusion for catheter-based erector spinae plane block on quality of recovery in thoracoscopic surgery: a single-centre randomised controlled trial. *Br J Anaesth.* 2024;133(4):874-881.

2. Taketa Y, Takayanagi Y, Irisawa Y, et al. Programmed intermittent bolus infusion vs. continuous infusion for erector spinae plane block in video-assisted thoracoscopic surgery: a double-blinded randomised controlled trial. *Eur J Anaesthesiol.* 2023;40(2):130-137.

3. Myles PS, Shulman MA, Reilly J, et al. Measurement of quality of recovery after surgery using the 15-item quality of recovery scale: a systematic review and meta-analysis. *Br J Anaesth.* 2022;128:1029-1039.

Paravertebral or pectoralis-II nerve blocks for non mastectomy breast surgery

29

Why this topic is important

Postoperative pain following breast surgery remains a significant challenge. Effective management is critical to improving recovery and minimizing opioid use. While thoracic paravertebral (PVB) blocks have long been the gold standard for regional anesthesia in breast surgery, newer fascial plane techniques, such as the pectoralis-II (PEC-II) block, have gained attention for their relative ease of administration and safety profile. A recent study by Gabriel et al. directly compares the analgesic effectiveness of these two blocks in patients undergoing nonmastectomy breast surgery-a subset of procedures that has received little focused investigation in the context of regional anesthesia. The findings can influence clinical decision-making and optimize pain management strategies.

Objectives of this update

- Compare the analgesic efficacy of PVB and PEC-II blocks regarding postoperative pain scores.

- Assess opioid consumption and recovery outcomes associated with these techniques.

- Identify patient and procedural factors that may guide block selection.

What is new

This randomized, observer-masked trial provides novel insights, including:

- Superior postoperative pain relief with PVB, with lower Numeric Rating Scale (NRS) pain scores in the recovery room compared to PEC-II.

- Reduced opioid requirements in patients receiving PVB, highlighting its opioid-sparing benefits.

- Contextualized findings that challenge previous studies, which have shown little difference between the blocks, by focusing specifically on nonmastectomy procedures.

Comparing the blocks

- Paravertebral block (PVB):

  ○ Involves injecting local anesthetic near the thoracic paravertebral space, providing somatic and sympathetic blockade (fig-1).

  ○ Demonstrated superior pain control across multiple studies, particularly for breast and thoracic surgeries.

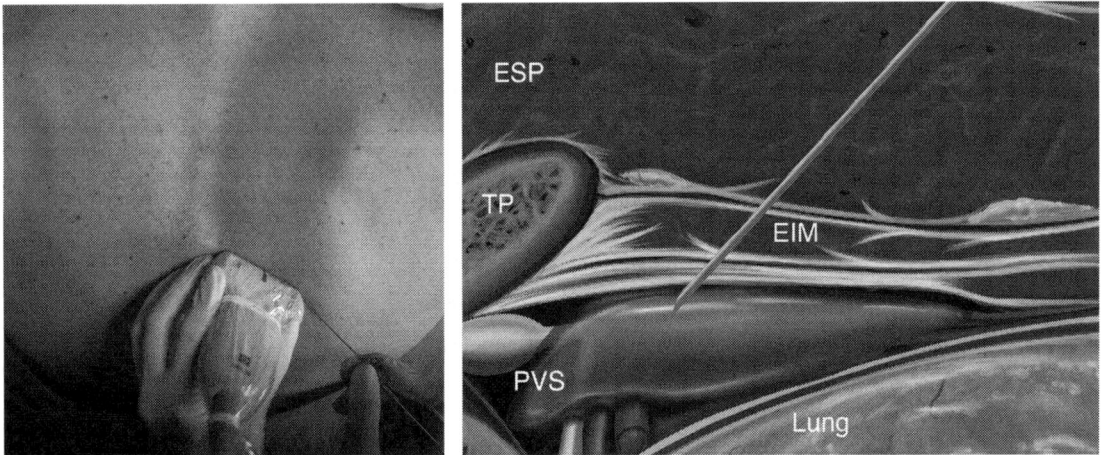

Fig-1. Reverse ultrasound anatomy of a paravertebral block when the transducer is placed in a transverse oblique orientation and in-plane approach. TP, transverse process; ESP, erector spinae muscles; PVS, paravertebral space; EIM, external intercostal muscle. Image taken from NYSORA LMS. https://nysoralms.com/

- Pectoralis-II block (PEC-II):

  ○ Targets the pectoral and serratus anterior fascial planes, blocking the medial and lateral pectoral nerves (fig-2).

  ○ Offers simpler placement and reduced risk of severe complications like pneumothorax.

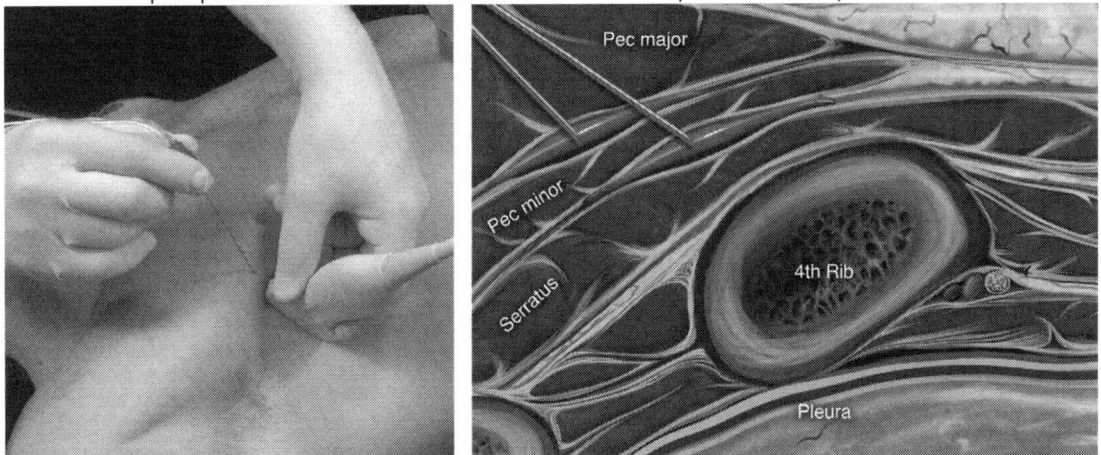

Fig-2. PEC II Reverse ultrasound anatomy. Needle insertion in-plane and local anesthetic spread 1) between the pectoralis major and minor muscles (PEC I) and 2) between the pectoralis minor and serratus anterior muscle. Image taken from NYSORA LMS. https://nysoralms.com/

Trial design and population

- Study structure:
  - Double-blinded, randomized design with 119 participants undergoing various nonmastectomy breast surgeries.
  - Equal distribution between PVB (n=59) and PEC-II (n=60) groups, ensuring comparability.

- Primary endpoints:
  - Pain scores in the recovery room using the NRS.
  - Total intraoperative and postoperative opioid consumption, measured in morphine milligram equivalents (MME).

Key results

- Pain scores:
  - Median recovery room pain scores were significantly lower with PVB (1.3) than PEC-II (3.3).
  - A greater percentage of PVB patients (39%) reported no pain versus PEC-II patients (18%).

- Opioid consumption:
  - Intraoperative and recovery room opioid use was lower in the PVB group (median 10.0 mg) versus the PEC-II group (17.5 mg).
  - A higher proportion of PVB patients required no additional opioids postoperatively (36% vs. 17%).

- Other outcomes:
  - PVB demonstrated prolonged analgesic effects, with lower pain scores and reduced oxycodone use even after recovery room discharge.
  - No block-related adverse events were reported, underscoring the safety of both techniques.

Clinical implications

- Pain management:
  - PVB provides superior pain relief and minimizes opioid use, making it the preferred choice for managing moderate to severe postoperative pain.

- Procedure selection:
  - PEC-II remains a viable alternative in cases where PVB is contraindicated, or practitioner expertise favors fascial plane techniques.

- Surgical considerations:
  - The findings highlight the need to tailor block choice based on the surgical site. PEC-II may offer better analgesia for axillary procedures, while PVB excels in breast-focused surgeries.

- Practical application:
  - Training programs should emphasize both techniques, allowing clinicians to choose the optimal approach based on patient and procedural needs.

Limitations

- Heterogeneous procedures: Inclusion of various nonmastectomy surgeries introduces variability, potentially affecting generalizability.

- Masking challenges: Differences in block placement techniques may have influenced patient perceptions.

- Incomplete enrollment: The study was terminated early, enrolling only 119 of the planned 150 participants.

Key takeaways

- ☑ PVB provides superior analgesia compared to PEC-II for nonmastectomy breast surgeries, with significantly lower pain scores and opioid requirements.

- ☑ PEC-II offers a safe and simpler alternative, which is particularly valuable in settings with limited resources or expertise in PVB placement.

- ☑ Block choice should consider surgical site, practitioner expertise, and patient-specific factors, with PVB being the preferred option for extensive breast procedures.

- ☑ Training in both techniques is essential to ensure flexibility and optimal patient outcomes.

Additional recommended reading

1. Gabriel RA, Curran BP, Swisher MW, et al. Paravertebral versus pectoralis-II nerve blocks for postoperative analgesia after nonmastectomy breast surgery: A randomized, controlled, observer-masked trial. *Anesthesiology.* 2024;141:1039-50.

2. Hussain N, Brull R, McCartney CJL, et al. Pectoralis-II myofascial block and analgesia in breast cancer surgery: A systematic review and meta-analysis. *Anesthesiology.* 2019;131:630-48.

3. Jin Z, Durrands T, Li R, et al. Pectoral block versus paravertebral block: A systematic review, meta-analysis, and trial sequential analysis. *Reg Anesth Pain Med.* 2020;45:727-32.

NYSORA

Serratus anterior plane block and early recovery from thoracoscopic lung resection

30

Why this topic is important

Minimally invasive thoracic surgeries, such as video-assisted thoracoscopic surgery (VATS) and robotic-assisted thoracoscopic surgery (RATS), are increasingly the standard of care for anatomic lung resections. These techniques reduce postoperative complications, facilitate faster recovery, and enhance overall outcomes compared to open thoracotomy. Despite these advancements, postoperative pain continues to challenge clinicians. The nature of thoracic pain is multifactorial, arising from local tissue trauma, nerve irritation, and visceral manipulation, compounded by intercostal and chest wall nociception. Effective pain management is vital for improving patient recovery, particularly in the context of enhanced recovery after surgery (ERAS) protocols.

ERAS protocols emphasize a multimodal analgesic approach to minimize reliance on opioids, thus mitigating side effects such as sedation, respiratory depression, nausea, and constipation. This opioid-sparing strategy is particularly relevant in the ongoing opioid crisis, which necessitates strategies to reduce acute and chronic opioid use after surgery. Regional anesthesia techniques, such as the serratus anterior plane (SAP) block, offer potential benefits as part of multimodal analgesia. The SAP block targets lateral cutaneous branches of the intercostal nerves, providing somatic pain relief for the chest wall. However, its utility as an adjunct in the management of thoracoscopic lung surgery pain remains debated.

This update focuses on recent evidence from a randomized controlled trial evaluating the SAP block's role in opioid reduction and early recovery following minimally invasive lung resection[1]. This research addresses knowledge gaps in how the SAP block compares to existing pain management strategies and its relevance in contemporary ERAS pathways.

Objectives of this update

- Evaluate the evidence for SAP block in reducing opioid consumption after thoracoscopic lung surgery.

- Summarize the effects of SAP block on secondary outcomes, including pain scores, respiratory function, recovery quality, and hospital stay.

- Integrate findings into clinical practice, emphasizing a multimodal approach to pain management.

What is new

A recent randomized, blinded, placebo-controlled trial examined the SAP block's efficacy in the setting of multimodal analgesia for minimally invasive thoracic lung surgery[1]. The study involved 99 patients undergoing elective anatomic lung resection at a single center. Patients were randomized to receive either a SAP block with bupivacaine, clonidine, and dexamethasone or a placebo block with saline.

The primary outcome was cumulative intravenous morphine equivalent consumption in the first 24 hours postoperatively. Secondary outcomes included pain scores at rest and during coughing, inspiratory effort, incidence of nausea or vomiting, Quality of Recovery (QoR-15) scores, and hospital length of stay. The findings provide nuanced insights into the SAP block's utility and limitations as part of ERAS protocols.

Detailed findings

Study design

The study was conducted within the framework of an institutional ERAS protocol. Key components of the perioperative management included intraoperative intravenous multimodal analgesics (fentanyl, dexamethasone, dexmedetomidine, acetaminophen, and ketorolac) and surgeon-administered intercostal nerve blocks. The SAP block was performed postoperatively using 40 mL of injectate containing bupivacaine 0.25%, clonidine, and dexamethasone in the intervention group, while the placebo group received saline injections in the same fascial plane.

Primary outcome: Opioid consumption

In the intention-to-treat analysis, the SAP block group showed a 32% reduction in 24-hour opioid use compared to the placebo group (median: 10.6 mg vs. 18.8 mg morphine equivalents, adjusted ratio 0.68). However, this difference did not reach statistical significance.

The as-treated analysis, which excluded logistical errors, demonstrated a significant 36% reduction in opioid use (median: 10.0 mg vs. 19.9 mg morphine equivalents, adjusted ratio 0.64). These findings suggest a modest opioid-sparing effect, particularly when the block is performed without deviations from the protocol.

Secondary outcomes

Pain scores:

- Pain at rest showed no significant differences between groups at any time point.
- The SAP block group significantly reduced pain with coughing, with a composite score improvement. This may reflect the block's ability to attenuate somatic pain from intercostal nerve irritation.

Inspiratory effort:

- Measured via incentive spirometry, postoperative inspiratory volumes were similar between groups on days 1 and 2.

Nausea and vomiting:

- The incidence of postoperative nausea or vomiting was not significantly different between the groups.

Quality of recovery (QoR-15):

- There was no significant improvement in QoR-15 scores in the SAP block group by postoperative day 7.

Length of hospital stay:

- The SAP block group had a 25% shorter hospital stay, though the difference was insignificant.

Safety:

- No block-related complications occurred, underscoring the SAP block's safety and feasibility as part of routine care.

Procedural considerations

The SAP block technique was performed quickly, averaging under 5 minutes, with ultrasound guidance ensuring precise delivery of the injectate into the fascial plane beneath the serratus anterior muscle. This straightforward approach offers several advantages:

- Ease of learning: Even anesthesiologists with limited ultrasound experience can perform the block with minimal training.

- Applicability in anticoagulated patients: The superficial location reduces the risk of bleeding complications compared to deeper blocks like paravertebral or epidural blocks.

- Favorable patient positioning: The block is easily administered in the lateral decubitus position used during thoracoscopic surgery.

The addition of clonidine and dexamethasone as adjuvants was aimed at prolonging block duration and enhancing analgesic efficacy.

Implications for practice

The findings highlight the SAP block's potential as a modestly effective adjunct in multimodal analgesia protocols for minimally invasive lung surgery. However, its benefits appear limited to certain metrics, such as opioid reduction and cough-related pain. These results suggest that while the SAP block can complement ERAS strategies, it should not replace other critical elements, such as intercostal nerve blocks and systemic analgesics.

When to consider the sap block?

1. Patient populations:

   - All patients can benefit from SAPB compared to no peripheral nerve block.

   - Benefits are particularly pronounced in patients at high risk for opioid-related side effects, such as the elderly or those with preexisting respiratory conditions.

   - Ideal for patients undergoing procedures where significant somatic chest wall pain is anticipated.

2. Institutional contexts:

   - Facilities with well-established ERAS pathways may benefit from incorporating SAP block as a low-risk addition to analgesia protocols.

   - Settings where alternative regional techniques (e.g., thoracic epidural or paravertebral blocks) are contraindicated.

Key takeaways

☑ The SAP block modestly reduces opioid consumption in thoracoscopic lung surgery but does not consistently improve secondary recovery outcomes.

☑ It is a safe, easy-to-perform technique that fits well within ERAS protocols, especially for patients where opioid reduction is a priority.

☑ The block's benefits are most pronounced for managing cough-associated pain.

☑ Integration into practice should be context-dependent, considering institutional resources and patient-specific factors.

Additional recommended reading

1. Jackson JC, Tan KS, Pedoto A, et al. Effects of serratus anterior plane block on early recovery from thoracoscopic lung resection: A randomized, blinded, placebo-controlled trial. *Anesthesiology*. 2024;141(6):1065-1074.

2. Blanco R, Parras T, McDonnell JG, Prats-Galino A. Serratus plane block: A novel ultrasound-guided thoracic wall nerve block. *Anaesthesia*. 2013;68:1107-13.

3. Kim DH, Oh YJ, Lee JG, et al. Efficacy of ultrasound-guided serratus plane block on postoperative quality of recovery and analgesia after video-assisted thoracic surgery: A randomized, triple-blind, placebo-controlled study. *Anesth Analg*. 2018;126:1353-61.

Serratus anterior plane block or paravertebral block in VATS

31

Why this topic is important

Postoperative pain control is a critical component of recovery following thoracic surgery, especially with the increasing use of Video-Assisted Thoracoscopic Surgery (VATS). Effective pain management reduces complications, such as pneumonia, improves patient satisfaction, and accelerates recovery. Inadequate pain control can lead to higher opioid consumption and prolonged hospital stays, undermining the goals of enhanced recovery protocols. Two regional anesthesia techniques, the Paravertebral Block (PVB) and the Serratus Anterior Plane Block (SAPB), are increasingly used in this context. Understanding their relative efficacy and the potential benefits of combining these techniques is essential for optimizing perioperative care.

Objectives of this update

- Review the role of PVB and SAPB in managing pain after VATS.

- Assess the effectiveness of these techniques alone and in combination.

- Evaluate the impact of these blocks on opioid consumption, pain intensity, and recovery.

- Provide evidence-based recommendations for anesthesia providers managing VATS patients

What is new

This update summarizes the findings from a recent double-blind, randomized trial comparing PVB, SAPB, and their combination in patients undergoing VATS[1]. While PVB is traditionally favored, SAPB presents a simpler, ultrasound-guided alternative that may better address anterior chest wall pain. Combining the two may provide comprehensive coverage but requires further validation. This update includes key outcomes, such as pain intensity at rest and during coughing, opioid use, and long-term pain control.

Comparison of block techniques

1. Paravertebral block (PVB) (fig-1)

   a. Anatomy and mechanism: It targets the thoracic intercostal nerves, providing effective pain relief for thoracic surgery by blocking multiple spinal nerves. It is performed at the T5-T6 level and is traditionally seen as a replacement for epidural analgesia.

   b. Advantages: Broad, reliable coverage of posterior and lateral chest wall pain.

   c. Challenges: Limited efficacy for anterior chest wall pain. Deep anatomical target and may be technically challenging in patients with poor ultrasound visibility.

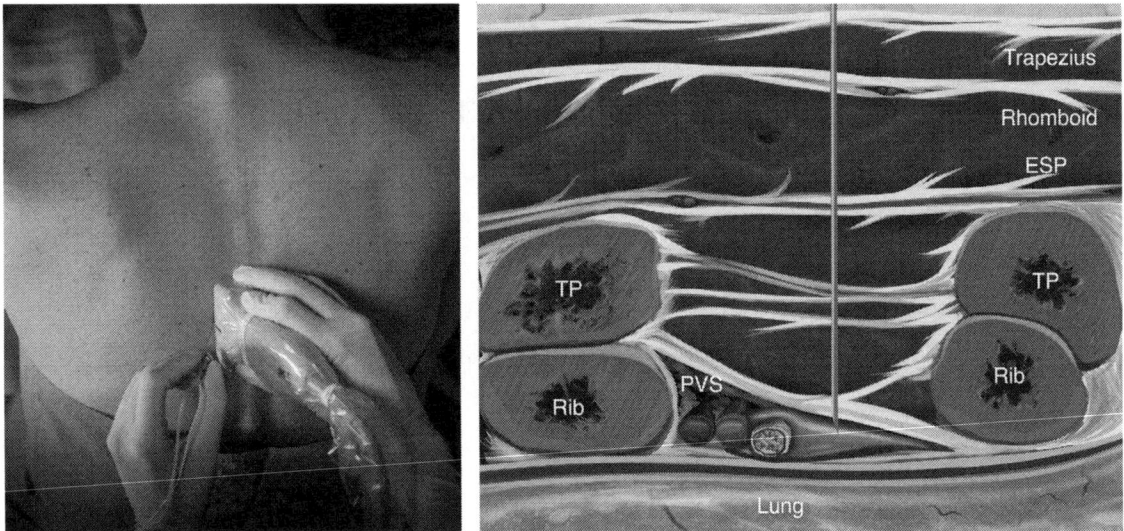

Fig-1. Reverse ultrasound anatomy of a paravertebral block when the transducer is placed in a sagittal orientation and an out-of-plane approach. TP, transverse process; PVS, paravertebral space; ESP, erector spinae muscles.
Image taken from NYSORA LMS. https://nysoralms.com/

2. Serratus anterior plane block (SAPB) (fig-2)

   a. Anatomy and mechanism: Focuses on the lateral branches of intercostal nerves by injecting anesthetic into the plane between the serratus anterior muscle and the rib. Provides good coverage of the anterior chest wall.

   b. Advantages: Simpler to perform with a superficial target, easier ultrasound visualization, and fewer technical challenges.

   c. Challenges: It is limited in its coverage of the posterior chest wall, which could leave portions of the surgical field inadequately anesthetized.

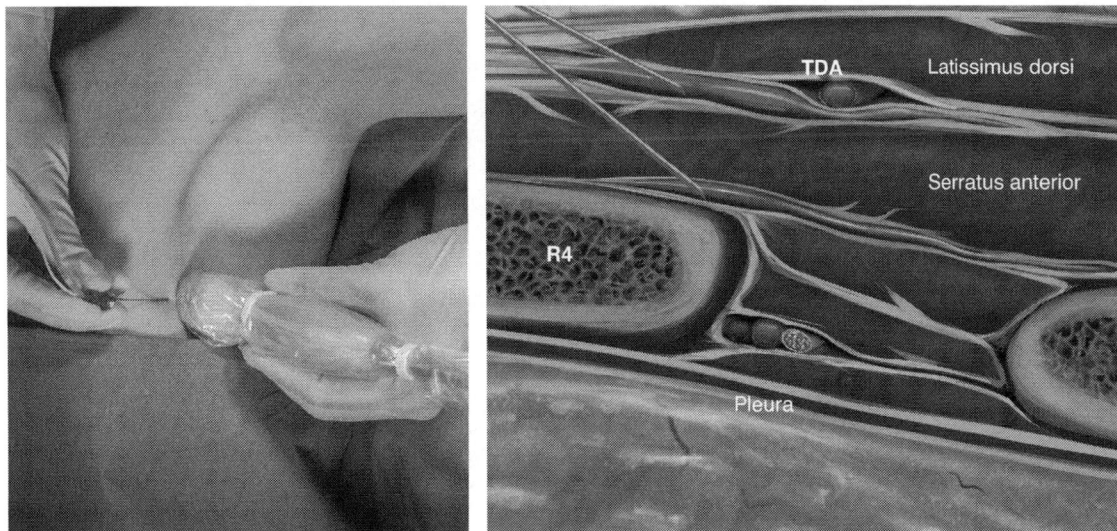

Fig-2. Reverse ultrasound anatomy of a serratus anterior plane block. Needle insertion in-plane with local anesthetic spread in option 1 (between latissimus dorsi and serratus anterior) or option 2 (underneath the serratus anterior muscle). TDA, thoracodorsal artery; R4, fourth rib. Image taken from NYSORA LMS. https://nysoralms.com/

3. Combination of PVB + SAPB

   a. Rationale: Combining the blocks aims to provide more comprehensive analgesia by covering both anterior and posterior chest walls. The hypothesis is that this would decrease opioid use and improve overall pain scores.

Study findings: Thoroascopic trial

The THORACOSOPIC trial evaluated the efficacy of PVB alone, SAPB alone, and the combination in patients undergoing elective VATS lung resection. A total of 156 patients were randomized into three groups: PVB, SAPB, and PVB + SAcombination of SAPB + PVB showed a trend toward lower pain scores, especially at rest and during coughing, though not immediately upon PACU admission.

- Opioid use: Opioid consumption was lower in the combination group than in individual blocks but did not reach statistical significance. This suggests a potential benefit in reducing opioid requirements but warrants further investigation.

- Pain trajectory: Compared to the single-block groups, the combined group had a faster decrease in pain intensity from PACU admission through hospital discharge.

Postoperative complications and long-term pain

- Hospital stays and rates of pneumonia did not differ significantly between groups.

- Neuropathic pain assessed at six months postoperatively was similar across all groups, indicating that none of the techniques conferred a long-term benefit in preventing chronic pain syndromes.

Comparison of PVB, SAPB, and combination techniques.

Parameter	PVB	SAPB	PVB + SAPB
Target area	Thoracic intercostal nerves	Lateral intercostal nerves	Combined anterior and posterior chest walls
Ease of placement	More difficult, deep structure	Easier, superficial placement	Moderate, combines both
Coverage	Posterior/lateral chest wall	Anterior chest wall	Comprehensive chest coverage
Challenges	Technical, deep structure	Limited posterior coverage	More time-consuming
Effectiveness in study[1]	Moderate, no superior benefit	Moderate, no superior benefit	Faster pain reduction post-op
Opioid reduction	No significant reduction	No significant reduction	Possible reduction

Primary outcome: Pain on coughing in the PACU

- On admission to the post-anesthesia care unit (PACU), the groups had no significant differences in pain scores. Median VAS pain scores were 3 for the PVB group, 4 for the SAPB group, and 2 for the combination group.

- Conclusion: Neither PVB nor SAPB alone was superior immediately post-surgery.

Secondary outcome: Pain and opioid consumption

- Over the course of postoperative care, the *Comparison of PVB, SAPB, and combination techniques.*

Implications for practice

While the combination of PVB and SAPB may offer some benefits in terms of faster pain reduction and potential opioid-sparing effects, this trial does not definitively demonstrate superiority over either block used alone. Institutional preferences, patient-specific anatomical considerations, and the relative ease of block placement may guide the choice of block.

Limitations of the study

- Blocks were performed after induction without testing for success, potentially leading to variable efficacy, especially for PVB. In cases of inadequate analgesia, the technical simplicity of SAPB makes it a viable supplemental option unless factors such as subcutaneous air, chest tubes, or tachypnea are present.

- The study lacks pain mapping data, leaving the specific regions of chest wall pain (anterior, lateral, posterior) unaddressed.

- The SAPB was performed exclusively as a deep block in this study, though alternative techniques (e.g., superficial block) were not discussed.

- Cumulative opioid use differences were not statistically significant, suggesting marginal benefits from the combination approach.

- Technical variability: Block efficacy can be influenced by operator skill and patient anatomy

- Pain was measured at fixed time points. Addressing pain trajectories dynamically over time could clarify the mechanism behind the observed trends in pain reduction.

Key takeaways

☑ SAPB and PVB are similar in effectiveness in managing post-VATS pain. However, SAPB may be a preferable supplementary option when analgesia is insufficient after PVB, given its technical simplicity and the ability to perform it without repositioning the patient-except in cases involving subcutaneous air, chest tubes, or tachypnea.

☑ The combination of SAPB + PVB may reduce pain more quickly and decrease opioid use but is not clearly superior to either block alone.

☑ Both blocks should be considered part of a broader multimodal pain management strategy in thoracic surgery.

Additional recommended reading

1. Leviel F, Fourdrain A, Delatre F, et al. Serratus anterior plane block alone, paravertebral block alone and their combination in video-assisted thoracoscopic surgery: the THORACOSOPIC double-blind, randomized trial. *Eur J Cardiothorac Surg.* 2024;65(4):ezae082.

2. Feray S, Lubach J, Joshi GP, Bonnet F, Van de Velde M; PROSPECT Working Group *of the European Society of Regional Anaesthesia and Pain Therapy. PROSPECT guidelines for video-assisted thoracoscopic surgery: a systematic review and procedure-specific postoperative pain management recommendations. *Anaesthesia.* 2022;77(3):311-325.

3. Nair S, Gallagher H, Conlon N. Paravertebral blocks and novel alternatives. *BJA Educ.* 2020;20(5):158-165.

Intertransverse process block in major breast cancer surgery

32

Why this topic is important

Postoperative pain management is a significant concern for patients undergoing major breast cancer surgeries, particularly those involving implant-based primary breast reconstruction. Uncontrolled pain can lead to prolonged recovery times, increased opioid use, and a higher incidence of opioid-related side effects, such as nausea, vomiting, and sedation, which further delay ambulation and hospital discharge. Given the current focus on reducing opioid consumption and improving recovery outcomes, finding effective regional anesthesia techniques is crucial.

The intertransverse process (ITP) block is a promising modality developed to mimic the effects of the thoracic paravertebral block (TPVB), targeting the ventral rami of the thoracic spinal nerves while avoiding the epidural space. By doing so, the ITP block aims to provide effective analgesia for hemithoracic procedures, such as major breast cancer surgeries. However, there has been a lack of robust evidence regarding its efficacy in reducing postoperative pain and opioid consumption in this specific patient population. Understanding whether this block can provide clinically meaningful benefits is critical to improving postoperative care in breast cancer surgery.

Objectives of this update

- To present findings from a recent randomized, placebo-controlled clinical trial[1] evaluating the efficacy of the ITP block in major breast cancer surgery.

- To discuss the implications of these findings for clinical practice, particularly in terms of postoperative pain management strategies.

What is new

A 2024 study by Nielsen et al.[1] is the first to rigorously evaluate the impact of the ITP block in a randomized, placebo-controlled trial for patients undergoing unilateral subpectoral implant-based breast reconstruction. Contrary to prior assumptions, the study found that the ITP block did not significantly reduce opioid consumption within the first 24 hours postoperatively, nor did it result in any substantial clinical improvements compared to placebo. These findings provide a critical perspective on the role of the ITP block in breast cancer surgery, suggesting that it may not be as beneficial as previously thought for deep tissue procedures.

Study design

The study by Nielsen et al. included 36 female patients with breast cancer scheduled for unilateral subpectoral implant-based breast reconstruction. This type of surgery typically involves the removal of the breast tissue, complete dissection of the anterior fascia of the major pectoral muscle, and placement of a subpectoral implant. Despite the use of a standardized multimodal analgesic regimen (preoperative acetaminophen, celecoxib, gabapentin, dexamethasone, and dextromethorphan), patients undergoing this surgery often experience significant postoperative pain.

Participants were randomly assigned to receive either an active ITP block (0.5% ropivacaine) or a placebo block (isotonic saline) at the thoracic levels T2, T4, and T6. The block was administered preoperatively to reduce postoperative pain and opioid consumption. The primary outcome measured was total opioid consumption within the first 24 hours after surgery. Secondary outcomes included opioid use at specific time intervals, pain intensity, time to ambulation and discharge, patient satisfaction with block application, and opioid-related side effects.

Key findings

1. Opioid consumption: There was no significant reduction in opioid consumption between the two groups. The median opioid consumption was 75 mg (interquartile range [IQR] 45-135 mg) in the active group and 62.5 mg (IQR 30-115 mg) in the placebo group, with a p-value of 0.5. This suggests that the ITP block did not have a significant opioid-sparing effect in this patient population.

2. Pain scores: Pain intensity, measured using the Numeric Rating Scale (NRS), showed no significant differences between the active and placebo groups at various postoperative time points. While both groups reported similar pain levels at rest and during movement, these results challenge the effectiveness of the ITP block in managing postoperative pain following major breast cancer surgery.

3. Patient satisfaction: Interestingly, patient satisfaction with block application was significantly higher in the active group at T2 and T4 injection levels, indicating that patients preferred the sensation or perceived benefit of the active block. However, this increased satisfaction did not correlate with better pain control or reduced opioid use.

4. Secondary outcomes: The time to first ambulation, time to discharge, and quality of recovery (QoR-15) scores were similar between the two groups. In fact, the placebo group showed a slight improvement in QoR-15 scores at 24 hours postoperatively compared to the active group, although this difference was not clinically significant.

5. Opioid-related side effects: Both groups experienced similar rates of opioid-related side effects, such as nausea and vomiting, indicating that the ITP block did not reduce the incidence of these complications.

Clinical implications

The lack of significant benefit from the ITP block in this study challenges its use as a primary analgesic strategy in major breast cancer surgery. There are several potential reasons why the ITP block may not have performed as expected in this patient population:

- The complexity of surgical pain: The dissection of the anterior fascia of the major pectoral muscle, which is heavily innervated by the brachial plexus, generates substantial postoperative pain. The ITP block, which targets thoracic spinal nerves, may not adequately cover the pain pathways involved in this surgery, particularly those related to the pectoral nerves (C5-T1). This underscores the need for additional blocks, such as pectoral nerve blocks (PECs) or interpectoral plane blocks, to target these specific nerves.

- Postoperative drains: The placement of postoperative drains, which manage fluid buildup after surgery, may introduce a neuropathic pain component that the ITP block does not address. Drains often exit near the axillary line, which may contribute to prolonged discomfort not alleviated by thoracic blocks.

- Anatomical limitations: The study found no evidence of significant pleural displacement, a marker used to indicate effective block placement in thoracic paravertebral studies. This suggests that the ITP block may not have fully reached the thoracic paravertebral space in all cases, limiting its effectiveness.

These findings indicate that the ITP block, when used alone, is unlikely to provide adequate postoperative analgesia for patients undergoing major breast cancer surgery involving deep tissue manipulation. Clinicians should consider supplementing the ITP block with other regional anesthesia techniques that target the brachial plexus and pectoral nerves to improve pain control. For example, the interpectoral plane block or pectoralis nerve block (PEC block) could be combined with the ITP block to provide more comprehensive analgesia.

Additionally, the role of the ITP block in other surgical contexts, such as minor thoracic procedures or surgeries with less extensive tissue manipulation, warrants further investigation. The block may be more effective in procedures where the pain pathways are more superficial and do not involve complex nerve innervation like that of the pectoral muscles.

Pain management in breast surgery	
Step 1	**Assess surgery type** • **Major** breast reconstruction with subpectoral implant → Move to Step 2 • **Minor** thoracic surgery → Consider ITP block alone.
Step 2	**Evaluate pectoral nerve involvement** • **Yes** (pectoral muscle dissection involved) → Add PECs block or interpectoral plane block. • **No** → Proceed with the ITP block.
Step 3	Implement a **multimodal analgesia regimen** (acetaminophen, gabapentin, NSAIDs) and administer blocks before surgery.

Key takeaways

☑ The ITP block does not significantly reduce opioid consumption or improve clinical outcomes following major breast cancer surgery involving subpectoral implant placement.

☑ Postoperative pain related to the major pectoral muscle dissection requires additional blocks targeting the pectoral nerves (e.g., PECs or interpectoral plane blocks).

☑ Further investigation is warranted into the role of the ITP block in less complex thoracic surgeries or as part of a multimodal analgesic strategy.

☑ Patient satisfaction with block application was high, but this did not translate into better pain relief or reduced opioid use.

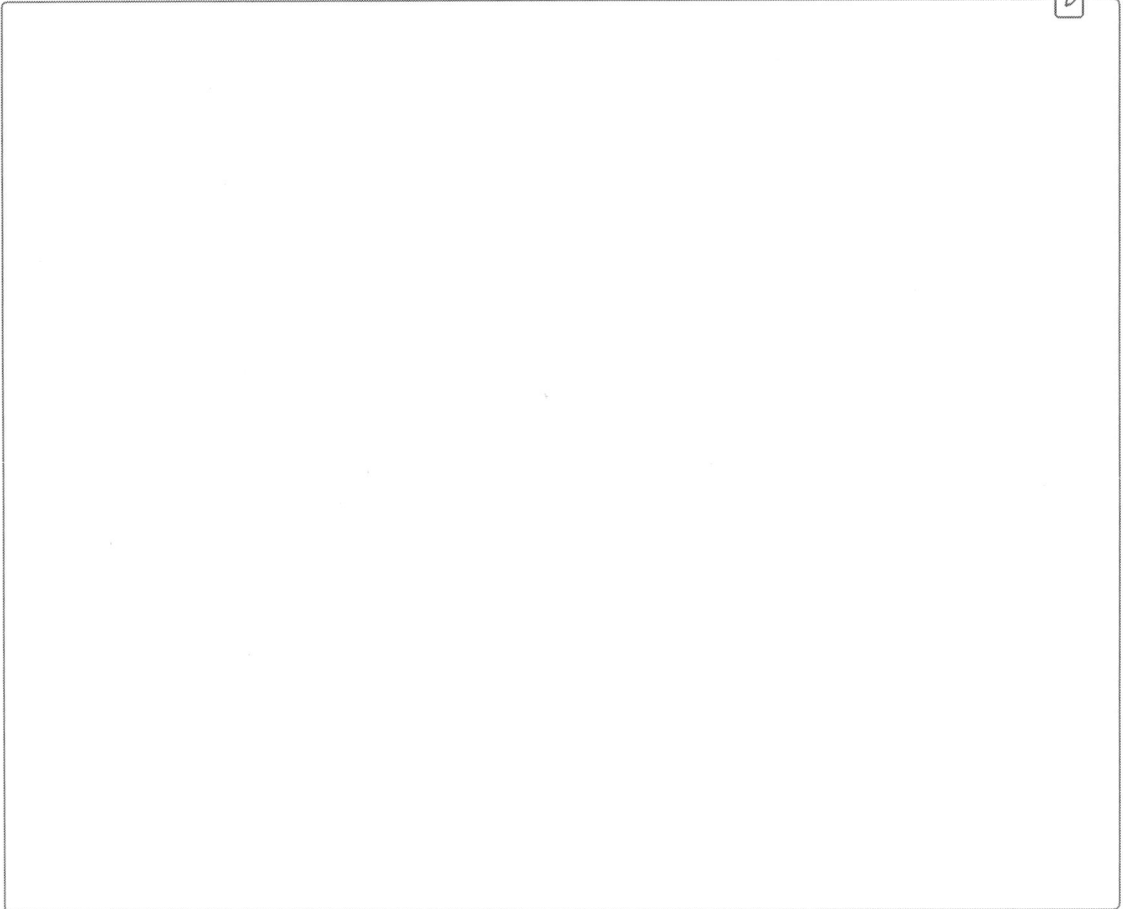

Additional recommended reading

1. Nielsen MV, Tanggaard K, Hansen LB, et al. Insignificant influence of the intertransverse process block for major breast cancer surgery: a randomized, blinded, placebo-controlled clinical trial. *Reg Anesth Pain Med.* 2024;49:10-16.

2. Aygun H, Kiziloglu I, Ozturk NK, et al. Use of ultrasound guided single shot costotransverse block in breast cancer surgery: a prospective, randomized, assessor-blinded controlled clinical trial. *BMC Anesthesiol.* 2022;22:110.

3. Zhang H, Qu Z, Miao Y, et al. Comparison between ultrasound-guided multi-injection intertransverse process and thoracic paravertebral blocks for major breast cancer surgery: a randomized non-inferiority trial. *Reg Anesth Pain Med.* 2023;48:161-6.

Analgesia after ESPB or surgical ICNB in VATS

33

Why this topic is important

Video-assisted thoracoscopic surgery (VATS) has gained popularity as a minimally invasive approach for thoracic procedures, offering reduced recovery times and smaller incisions. Despite these advantages, many patients undergoing VATS experience moderate to severe postoperative pain. Effective pain management is crucial to enhance recovery, reduce opioid use, and improve patient outcomes. Regional anesthesia techniques, including the ultrasound-guided erector spinae plane block (ESPB) and surgical intercostal nerve block (ICNB), have been used to manage pain after VATS. However, there is a limited direct comparison of their analgesic efficacy. This update aims to provide insight into the latest randomized controlled trial[1] that compares ESPB and ICNB to guide clinicians in selecting the optimal pain management strategy for VATS patients.

Objectives of this update

- Compare the analgesic effectiveness of ultrasound-guided erector spinae plane block (ESPB) with a surgical intercostal nerve block (ICNB) following VATS.

- Review outcomes related to postoperative pain scores and opioid consumption over a 48-hour postoperative period.

- Highlight the differences in postoperative recovery, including quality of recovery, duration of chest tube drainage, and length of hospital stay.

- Based on recent evidence, provide clinical guidance for the routine use of regional anesthesia in VATS.

What is new

This update is based on a randomized, double-blind study of 100 patients undergoing VATS for lung tumor resection. It compared the analgesic effects of anesthesiologist-administered ESPB and surgeon-administered ICNB. Key findings:

- Both ESPB and ICNB provided similar postoperative pain relief at [1], 24, and 48 hours.

- ESPB had slightly higher but non-significant morphine use over 48 hours.

- ICNB reduced oral rescue analgesic use, though not significantly.

- Both techniques had comparable outcomes for recovery, chest tube drainage, and hospital stay length.

Overview of regional anesthesia techniques in VATS

1. Ultrasound-guided erector spinae plane block (ESPB)

The ESPB, introduced in 2016, is a relatively new regional anesthesia technique for managing thoracic pain. It involves injecting a local anesthetic between the erector spinae muscle and the transverse process of the thoracic vertebra, which spreads across multiple levels, providing effective pain relief for thoracic surgeries. ESPB is considered easier to perform than other blocks, such as the paravertebral block, making it a practical option for VATS procedures.

- Procedure: In the study, ESPB was performed at the T5 vertebra level, and 20 mL of 0.5% levobupivacaine was injected.

- Advantages: The ESPB is ultrasound-guided, allowing the anesthesiologist to visualize the needle placement and the spread of the local anesthetic in real-time.

2. Surgical intercostal nerve block (ICNB)

ICNB has been widely used in thoracic surgery and can be administered by the surgeon under direct visualization during VATS. The block involves injecting a local anesthetic around the intercostal nerves at the surgical site, providing targeted pain relief.

- Procedure: In the study, the surgeon performed ICNB, injecting 4 mL of 0.5% levobupivacaine into the intercostal spaces, two above and two below the surgical incision, for a total of 20 mL.

- Advantages: ICNB is performed under direct thoracoscopic visualization, ensuring accurate placement of the local anesthetic.

Primary outcomes

3. Pain scores

Postoperative pain was assessed using a 10-cm visual analog scale (VAS), with scores recorded at 1 hour, 24 hours, and 48 hours after surgery. Both ESPB and ICNB demonstrated low pain scores (below 4) at all time points, and there was no statistically significant difference between the two groups:

- At 24 hours (peak pain intensity), the dynamic VAS scores were:

  ○ ESPB group: Median VAS 3.0

  ○ ICNB group: Median VAS 3.6

These findings suggest that both ESPB and ICNB provide effective pain relief, maintaining VAS scores within an acceptable range for postoperative comfort.

4. Morphine consumption

Morphine consumption was used as a secondary measure of analgesic effectiveness. While there was a trend toward higher morphine consumption in the ESPB group, the differences were not statistically significant:

- 48-hour morphine consumption:

  ○ ESPB group: Median 3 mg

  ○ ICNB group: Median 0 mg

Secondary outcomes

1. Quality of Recovery

Patient recovery was evaluated using the Quality of Recovery-15 (QoR-15) questionnaire within 24 hours post-surgery. There was no significant difference between the two groups:

- QoR-15 scores:

  ○ ESPB group: Median 117

  ○ ICNB group: Median 113

Both ESPB and ICNB provided good quality of recovery scores, indicating that either technique can support rapid recovery following VATS.

2. Chest tube drainage and hospital stay

The duration of chest tube drainage and hospital stay are important markers of recovery in thoracic surgery. The study found no significant differences between the two groups in these metrics:

- Chest tube drainage duration: Median of 2 days in both groups.

- Hospital stay: Median of 5.5-6 days in both groups.

These results indicate that both ESPB and ICNB are equally effective in facilitating early recovery after VATS.

Discussion and clinical implications

This study provides robust evidence supporting using both ESPB and ICNB for postoperative analgesia in VATS. Despite some minor differences in morphine consumption and oral rescue analgesic use, both techniques were comparable in terms of pain relief, recovery, and secondary outcomes. Based on these findings:

- ICNB offers a practical, surgeon-administered option for regional analgesia in VATS. Since it is performed under direct visualization during the surgery, ICNB can be easily incorporated into the surgical workflow, particularly in centers with limited anesthesiology resources.

- ESPB remains a valuable tool, particularly when surgeon-administered blocks are not feasible.

Considerations for Clinical Practice:

- For minor thoracic resections, such as wedge resection, where pain intensity and duration may be lower, ICNB may be favored for its ease and convenience.

- For more extensive thoracic surgeries or cases with a high risk of pleural adhesions, ESPB may offer advantages.

Limitations

Several limitations should be considered when interpreting the results of this study:

1. Small sample size: While the study enrolled 100 patients, larger trials may be necessary to detect subtle differences between ESPB and ICNB.

2. No sensory testing: The study did not include preoperative or postoperative sensory testing to determine the exact dermatomal coverage of the nerve blocks.

3. Single-shot blocks: Both ESPB and ICNB were administered as single-shot blocks. Future studies should explore the benefits of continuous catheter techniques, especially for ESPB, which has been shown to provide prolonged analgesia when used with catheters.

Key takeaways

- ☑ Both ESPB and ICNB provide effective pain control following VATS, with comparable pain scores and recovery outcomes.

- ☑ ICNB is a convenient option as it can be performed by the surgeon during VATS, making it practical for minor surgeries.

- ☑ ESPB may offer extended pain relief and can be administered by an anesthesiologist using ultrasound guidance.

- ☑ Clinicians should individualize their choice of block based on the surgical complexity, availability of anesthesia resources, and patient-specific factors.

Additional recommended reading

1. Sung CS, Wei TJ, Hung JJ, et al. Comparisons in analgesic effects between ultrasound-guided erector spinae plane block and surgical intercostal nerve block after video-assisted thoracoscopic surgery: A randomized controlled trial. *J Clin Anesth.* 2024;95:111448.

2. Forero M, Adhikary SD, Lopez H, Tsui C, Chin KJ. The erector spinae plane block: a novel analgesic technique in thoracic neuropathic pain. *Reg Anesth Pain Med.* 2016;41:621-7.

3. Gams P, Bitenc M, Danojevic N, et al. Erector spinae plane block versus intercostal nerve block for postoperative analgesia in lung cancer surgery. *Radiol Oncol.* 2023;57:364-70.

Posterior QLB or Intrathecal morphine in cesarean section

34

Why this topic is important

Postoperative pain management for cesarean sections (CS) is essential for optimal maternal recovery and neonatal care. Effective analgesia not only improves patient comfort but also plays a critical role in preventing complications like chronic pain, prolonged opioid use, and delayed maternal-infant bonding. Traditional analgesia often includes intrathecal morphine (ITM), which, though effective, has notable side effects, including nausea, vomiting, and pruritus. These adverse effects can limit morphine's suitability for some patients, especially those sensitive to opioids.

As an alternative, regional anesthesia techniques like the quadratus lumborum block (QLB) have gained attention for their potential to reduce postoperative pain with fewer side effects. A recent study by Giral et al.[1] offers new insights into using the posterior approach for QLB (PQLB) with ropivacaine, examining its efficacy and safety compared to ITM for postoperative analgesia in scheduled CS. The PQLB targets the posterior fascial plane of the QL muscle, deep to the middle layer of the thoracolumbar fascia (fig-1).

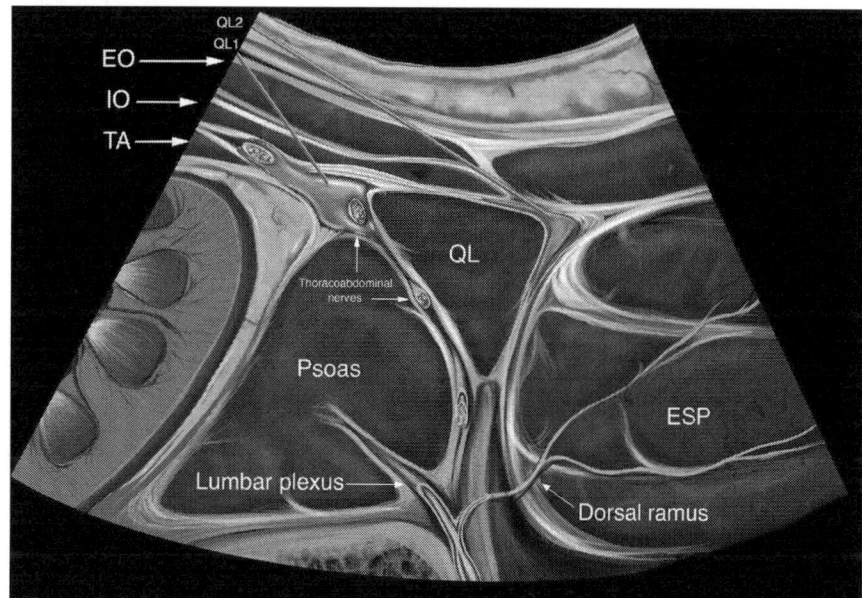

Fig-1. Reverse ultrasound anatomy with needle insertion points for a posterior quadratus lumborum block (also known as the QL2 block). Ideal local anesthetic spread (blue area) for a QL2 block - posterior to the QL muscle. EO, external oblique; IO, internal oblique; TA, transversus abdominis; QL, quadratus lumborum; ESP, erector spinae muscles.
Image taken from NYSORA LMS. https://nysoralms.com/

By exploring whether PQLB offers comparable pain control to ITM while reducing side effects, this research highlights an innovative approach to improve patient outcomes and experiences in cesarean section recovery.

Objectives of this update

- Evaluate analgesic efficacy: To assess whether PQLB with ropivacaine provides comparable pain relief to ITM in the first 24 hours after CS.

- Compare side effects: To understand differences in adverse effects between ITM and PQLB, particularly opioid-related pruritus and nausea.

- Inform clinical practice: To discuss practical implications of PQLB as an alternative to ITM, especially in cases of morphine sensitivity or contraindication, contributing to patient-centered analgesic strategies.

What is new

- Comparable analgesia: PQLB and ITM demonstrated similar effectiveness in managing pain during the first 24 hours post-CS, with no significant differences in cumulative morphine use.

- Reduced side effects with PQLB: PQLB resulted in significantly fewer instances of pruritus and nausea than ITM, offering an option with a better safety profile for patients sensitive to opioids.

- Improved functional recovery: Patients who received PQLB showed enhanced recovery scores at 24 hours, indicating potential benefits for early mobilization and maternal-infant interactions.

Clinical study overview

Study methods & design

The study[1] was a randomized, blinded, controlled trial conducted on 104 patients scheduled for cesarean delivery under spinal anesthesia. Patients were randomly assigned to receive either ITM or bilateral PQLB with ropivacaine. To ensure unbiased data, participants and evaluators were blinded to treatment allocation.

Primary outcome: The study's main endpoint was the cumulative intravenous morphine requirement over the first 24 hours post-surgery, as measured through patient-controlled analgesia (PCA).

Secondary outcomes: Additional outcomes included cumulative morphine use at multiple time points (6, 12, 24, and 48 hours), pain levels at rest and during movement, functional recovery as measured by the Obstetric Quality of Recovery (ObsQoR-11) questionnaire, and adverse events.

Procedure details

- ITM group: This group received a single dose of 0.1 mg/mL intrathecal morphine, administered as part of spinal anesthesia.

- PQLB group: Participants in this group received 140 mg ropivacaine, injected bilaterally into the posterior quadratus lumborum space under ultrasound guidance, following standard protocols for targeting the abdominal innervation regions relevant to cesarean section incisions.

Statistical methods

Power analysis indicated a sample size of 104 to detect meaningful differences in morphine consumption, while statistical tests included repeated measurements, Student's t-tests, and Mann-Whitney U tests for data analysis.

Results

Primary endpoint - 24-hour morphine consumption

The cumulative morphine requirement at 24 hours did not differ significantly between groups. The PQLB group required an average of 13.7 mg, while the ITM group required 11.1 mg. This result suggests that both PQLB and ITM offer comparable analgesic effectiveness during the critical first day of postoperative recovery.

Secondary outcomes

- Pain Scores: Across most time points, pain scores were similar between groups. However, dynamic pain (pain during movement or coughing) was lower in the PQLB group at 6 hours postoperatively, suggesting an initial advantage for PQLB in managing activity-related discomfort.

- Functional Recovery (ObsQoR-11): Recovery scores at 24 hours were higher in the PQLB group, indicating that patients in this group were more comfortable and mobile earlier in the postoperative period. By 48 hours, scores had leveled out between the groups.

- Adverse Effects: ITM was associated with a higher frequency of pruritus (60%) compared to PQLB (2%). Other opioid-related side effects, like nausea, were rare due to prophylactic antiemetics but still noted predominantly in the ITM group.

Discussion

Analgesic efficacy

Both ITM and PQLB proved to be effective in controlling pain after cesarean delivery, with similar morphine consumption in the first 24 hours. Although no overall difference in pain control was found, PQLB showed benefits for activity-related pain at the 6-hour mark. This advantage in dynamic pain management aligns with previous findings indicating that regional blocks like PQLB may better address pain associated with movement, a crucial factor for early mobilization and postoperative recovery.

Functional recovery and early mobilization

Enhanced ObsQoR-11 scores in the PQLB group at 24 hours postoperatively suggest an earlier return to physical comfort and independence. Patients in this group were more likely to mobilize, potentially contributing to earlier bonding with their newborns, which is particularly beneficial in the cesarean recovery context. By promoting more rapid engagement in daily activities, PQLB might facilitate early discharge, reduce hospital stays, and support maternal-infant interaction.

Side effect profile

The markedly lower incidence of pruritus in the PQLB group highlights one of its primary advantages over ITM. Pruritus is a common side effect of opioid administration and can significantly detract from patient comfort. In contrast, regional anesthesia with ropivacaine in the PQLB group showed a minimal incidence of pruritus and similar rates of nausea, managed effectively with standard antiemetic prophylaxis. Given this profile, PQLB offers a safer option for patients who are either sensitive to opioids or wish to minimize exposure.

Technical considerations and feasibility

PQLB is a technically demanding procedure that requires ultrasound guidance and an experienced anesthetist to ensure precise placement within the quadratus lumborum space. This study used a posterior approach to target abdominal innervation relevant to cesarean incisions, known for effective spread to abdominal parietal and visceral nerves. However, challenges include patient repositioning to access both sides and increased resource needs for equipment and personnel.

Given these requirements, PQLB may not be feasible in all clinical settings. The simplicity and rapid application of ITM in the same syringe as spinal anesthesia may be more accessible in settings with fewer resources or less anesthetic expertise. Nonetheless, when available, PQLB offers a high-value alternative with reduced side effects, particularly useful for patients with opioid sensitivity.

Comparison of analgesic efficacy and safety profiles.

Parameter	PQLB	ITM
Analgesic effectivesness	Similar 24-hour morphine use; better for dynamic pain at 6 hours	Similar overall effectiveness
Time to first morphine request	+/- 9 hours	+/- 5 hours
Pruritus	2%	60%
Nausea and vomiting	Low (with prophylaxis)	Low (with prophylaxis)
Functional recovery at 24 hours	Improved (higher ObsQoR-11 scores)	Lower ObsQoR-11 scores
Technical feasibility	Requires ultrasound and expertise	Simpler and faster

Key takeaways

☑ Comparable pain control: PQLB with ropivacaine offers similar pain relief to ITM within the first 24 hours after cesarean section, making it a viable alternative for effective postoperative analgesia.

☑ Reduced adverse effects: PQLB had significantly less pruritus compared to ITM, which may improve patient comfort and tolerance, particularly for opioid-sensitive patients.

☑ Enhanced functional recovery: Early mobilization and comfort were superior in the PQLB group at 24 hours, promoting earlier bonding with the newborn and potentially supporting shorter hospital stays.

☑ Extended time to PCA request: The time to first PCA morphine request was longer for patients in the PQLB group, indicating an extended duration of initial pain relief.

☑ Practical limitations: While PQLB requires more expertise and resources, it is an effective alternative in settings where skilled anesthetists and ultrasound guidance are available, especially beneficial for patients with high opioid sensitivity.

Additional recommended reading

1. Giral, T., Delvaux, B. V., Huynh, D., et al. "Posterior Quadratus Lumborum Block vs Intrathecal Morphine Analgesia After Scheduled Cesarean Section: A Prospective, Randomized, Controlled Study." *Reg Anesth Pain Med* 2024.

2. Singh, N. P., Makkar, J. K., Koduri, S., et al. "Efficacy of Different Approaches of Quadratus Lumborum Block for Postoperative Analgesia After Cesarean Delivery: A Bayesian Network Meta-analysis." *Clin J Pain* 2023;39:634-42.

3. Ryu, C., Choi, G. J., Jung, Y. H., et al. "Postoperative Analgesic Effectiveness of Peripheral Nerve Blocks in Cesarean Delivery: A Systematic Review and Network Meta-Analysis." *J Pers Med* 2022;12:634.

Anterior QLB and the immune response after laparoscopic colon cancer surgery

35

Why this topic is important

Surgery, while curative in many cancer cases, induces systemic inflammatory and immune responses that can affect recovery and long-term outcomes. Colorectal cancer surgery, in particular, is associated with significant physiological stress, leading to altered immune cell function and cytokine production. These changes can contribute to perioperative complications and potentially facilitate metastatic progression.

Regional anesthesia techniques, such as the anterior quadratus lumborum (QL) block (fig-1), offer benefits for postoperative pain management, reducing opioid consumption, and possibly modulating surgical stress responses. However, the extent to which the anterior QL block influences systemic immune changes has remained unclear. Given the growing interest in optimizing perioperative care to enhance recovery and potentially improve oncological outcomes, exploring the immune-modulatory effects of regional anesthesia is highly relevant.

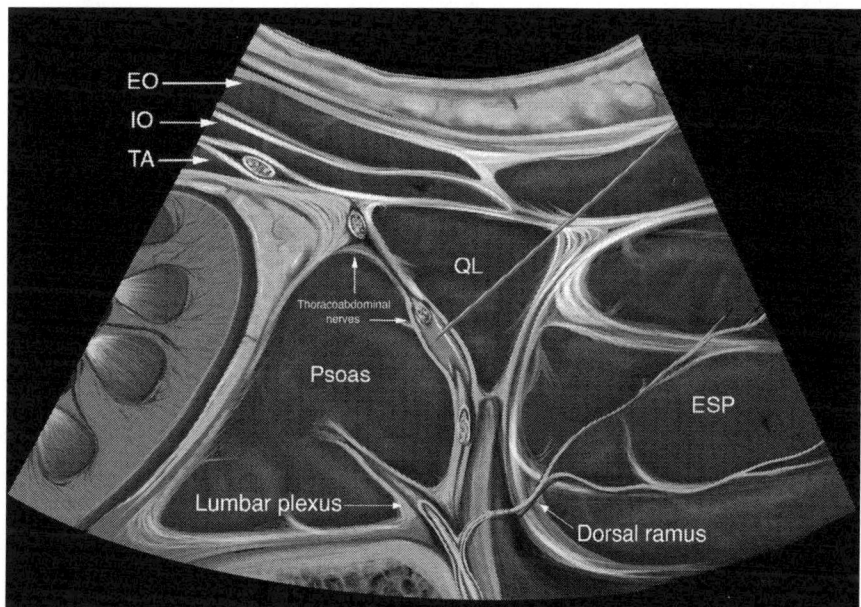

Fig-1. Reverse ultrasound anatomy with needle insertion in-plane for an anterior quadratus lumborum (QL3) block. Ideal local anesthetic distribution (blue) on the anterior aspect of the QL muscle. EO, external oblique; IO, internal oblique; TA, transversus abdominis; QL, quadratus lumborum; ESP, erector spinae muscles. Image taken from NYSORA LMS. https://nysoralms.com/

This update examines findings from a substudy of a randomized controlled trial assessing the impact of the anterior QL block on systemic immune responses in laparoscopic hemicolectomy patients[1].

Objectives of this update

- Evaluate the effect of anterior QL block on the immune system's transcriptional and cytokine responses post-surgery.

- Highlight its role in enhanced recovery protocols for colorectal cancer patients.

- Discuss the clinical implications of regional anesthesia in modulating surgical stress and immune function.

What is new

This substudy by Balsevicius et al. utilized gene expression profiling and cytokine assays to assess systemic immune changes in 22 patients randomized to receive anterior QL block with ropivacaine or placebo during laparoscopic colectomy.

Key findings:

- The anterior QL block did not alter gene expression in circulating immune cells.

- No significant changes were observed in plasma cytokine levels or predicted immune cell populations.

- Immune activation pathways remained unaffected postoperatively.

Detailed findings

Study design

This substudy was embedded within a double-blind, randomized controlled trial involving 22 patients undergoing laparoscopic hemicolectomy for colon cancer. Patients were randomized to receive either a bilateral anterior QL block with ropivacaine (30 mL of 0.375% per side) or isotonic saline placebo. Blood samples were collected preoperatively and 24 hours postoperatively for molecular analyses.

Primary outcomes

1. Gene expression:

   ◦ A targeted panel of 750 immune-related genes revealed no significant differences in transcriptional profiles between groups.

   ◦ Hierarchical clustering and principal component analysis showed no separation by treatment, suggesting no systemic immune modulation.

2. Cytokine levels:

   ◦ Plasma levels of 17 cytokines representing various immune pathways (e.g., type 1, type 2, type 17 responses, regulatory responses) showed no significant changes postoperatively in either group.

3. Immune cell composition:

   ◦ Inferred immune cell populations from transcriptomic data (e.g., T cells, NK cells, granulocytes) did not differ between groups.

4. Immune activation assays:

   ◦ Ex vivo stimulation of whole blood with immune activators (e.g., LPS, anti-CD3/CD28) demonstrated robust cytokine responses but no differences between treatment arms.

Implications for practice

Pain management without immune modulation

The anterior QL block is effective for postoperative pain relief and reducing opioid consumption, as demonstrated in other studies. However, its lack of impact on systemic immune responses indicates that it does not alter the inflammatory stress associated with surgery. This suggests its utility lies primarily in analgesia rather than immune modulation.

Patient safety and clinical feasibility

- Safety profile: The anterior QL block did not adversely affect immune function, making it a safe option for perioperative pain management in immunocompromised or cancer patients.

- ERAS protocol integration: The block can be integrated into enhanced recovery protocols without concerns about compromising immune response, providing targeted pain relief while maintaining systemic physiological stability.

Challenges and limitations

1. Sample size:

   ○ The small cohort size may limit the ability to detect subtle immune effects. Larger trials are needed to validate these findings.

2. Baseline immune variability:

   ○ Differences in patient baseline immune status (e.g., cancer stage, comorbidities) were not fully addressed, which could influence immune responses.

3. Limited assessment duration:

   ○ Immune responses were only assessed up to 24 hours postoperatively, missing potential delayed effects.

4. Concurrent analgesic techniques:

   ○ Standard wound infiltration analgesia, part of the ERAS protocol, may have masked any independent immune effects of the anterior QL block.

Key takeaways

☑ The anterior QL block relieves effective postoperative pain without altering systemic immune responses.

☑ It is a safe and feasible addition to enhanced recovery protocols for laparoscopic colorectal surgery.

☑ Its primary benefit lies in analgesia, with no evidence of immune modulation based on current findings.

Additional recommended reading

1. Balsevicius L, Urbano PCM, Hasselager RP, et al. Effect of anterior quadratus lumborum block with ropivacaine on the immune response after laparoscopic surgery in colon cancer: A substudy of a randomized clinical trial. *Reg Anesth Pain Med.* 2024;49:805-814.

2. Ackerman RS, Luddy KA, Icard BE, et al. The effects of anesthetics and perioperative medications on immune function: A narrative review. *Anesth Analg.* 2021;133:676-689.

3. Dockrell L, Buggy DJ. The role of regional anaesthesia in the emerging subspecialty of onco-anaesthesia: A state-of-the-art review. *Anaesthesia.* 2021;76(Suppl 1):148-159.

ESPB with intercostal nerve cryoablation for Nuss procedures

36

Why this topic is important

Pectus excavatum (PE), the most common anterior chest wall deformity, often requires surgical correction via the minimally invasive Nuss procedure. While effective, this technique is associated with significant postoperative pain, necessitating robust analgesic strategies. Historically, pain management has relied on opioids, patient-controlled analgesia, neuraxial blocks, and surgical cryoablation of intercostal nerves.

The erector spinae plane (ESP) block, a novel regional anesthesia technique, has demonstrated efficacy in reducing pain and opioid use in thoracic surgeries. Combining ESP blocks with cryoablation has the potential to optimize perioperative pain control, reduce opioid-related side effects, and shorten hospital stays. A recent study by Aranda-Valderrama et al. evaluates the combined use of these modalities in children undergoing the Nuss procedure, offering valuable insights for improving perioperative pathways.

Objectives of this update

- To assess the impact of combining ESP blocks with intercostal nerve cryoablation on postoperative opioid consumption and hospital length of stay (LOS).

- To determine whether the combined approach improves pain management compared to cryoablation alone.

- To evaluate the feasibility and safety of incorporating ESP blocks into the perioperative pathway for Nuss procedures.

What is new

This study of Aranda-Valderrama et al. 2024 provides the first direct comparison of cryoablation alone versus cryoablation combined with ESP blocks in pediatric patients undergoing the Nuss procedure. It highlights significant reductions in total opioid use and hospital LOS with the combined approach, without adverse events related to block placement.

Study findings

Methodology

- Design: Retrospective cohort study at a tertiary pediatric hospital.

- Participants: 40 pediatric patients undergoing the Nuss procedure, divided into two groups:

  - Cryo-only group: 20 patients receiving intercostal nerve cryoablation alone.

  - ESP + Cryo group: 20 patients receiving bilateral ESP blocks with intercostal nerve cryoablation.

- Interventions: ESP blocks were performed preoperatively under ultrasound guidance using 20 mL of 0.35% ropivacaine with clonidine at the T6 level.

- Outcomes: Primary outcomes were total opioid consumption (morphine milligram equivalents, MME) and hospital LOS. Secondary outcomes included pain scores, surgical time, and block-related adverse events.

Results

1. Opioid consumption

   - Total hospital opioid use was significantly lower in the ESP + Cryo group (median 0.60 MME/kg) compared to the Cryo-only group (median 1.15 MME/kg).

   - Opioid reduction was particularly notable on postoperative days (POD) 1 and 2, with a 60% reduction observed in the ESP + Cryo group.

2. Pain scores

   - No significant difference in median pain scores was observed between groups on POD 0-2, suggesting effective pain control with both techniques.

3. Hospital length of stay

   - The ESP + Cryo group had a shorter mean LOS (1.95 days) than the Cryo-only group (2.45 days).

   - 25% of patients in the ESP + Cryo group were discharged on POD 1, while all patients in the Cryo-only group were discharged on POD 2 or later.

4. Safety and feasibility

   - ESP block placement added an average of 12.5 minutes to the preoperative preparation time but did not delay surgical schedules.

   - No adverse events related to ESP block placement were reported.

Clinical implications

Bridging analgesia with ESP blocks

Cryoablation effectively relieves pain by inducing intercostal nerve paresthesia, but its onset is delayed, often requiring bridging analgesia in the immediate postoperative period. ESP blocks provide a non-opioid bridging solution, reducing opioid consumption and its associated side effects.

Optimizing discharge readiness

The shorter LOS observed in the ESP + Cryo group suggests that improved analgesia can accelerate functional recovery, facilitate early mobilization, and enhance discharge readiness. This aligns with enhanced recovery after surgery (ERAS) protocols.

Safety and accessibility

ESP blocks are technically simpler and carry a lower risk of complications than thoracic epidurals and paravertebral blocks, making them accessible to a broader range of anesthesia providers.

Limitations

- Retrospective design: The study design precludes randomization and control of confounding variables.

- Sample size: The small cohort size limits generalizability.

- Non-standardized analgesia: Variability in perioperative opioid regimens may influence results.

Key takeaways

- ☑ Combining ESP blocks with intercostal nerve cryoablation significantly reduces opioid consumption and hospital LOS in pediatric patients undergoing the Nuss procedure.

- ☑ Both techniques provide effective pain control, with ESP blocks serving as an opioid-sparing bridge during the delayed onset of cryoablation analgesia.

- ☑ The combined approach is safe, feasible, and aligns with ERAS protocols for early discharge and functional recovery.

- ☑ Further research is needed to optimize protocols and confirm findings in larger, randomized studies.

Additional recommended reading

1. Aranda-Valderrama P, Greenberg RS, Vecchione TM, et al. Combined erector spinae plane block with surgical intercostal nerve cryoablation for Nuss procedure is associated with decreased opioid use and length of stay. *Reg Anesth Pain Med.* 2024;49:248-253. doi:10.1136/rapm-2023-104407.

2. Santana L, Driggers J, Carvalho NF. Pain management for the Nuss procedure: comparison between erector spinae plane block, thoracic epidural, and control. *World J Pediatr Surg.* 2022;5:e000418.

3. Bliss DP, Strandness TB, Derderian SC, et al. Ultrasound-guided erector spinae plane block versus thoracic epidural analgesia: postoperative pain management after Nuss repair for pectus excavatum. *J Pediatr Surg.* 2022;57:207-212.

Superficial parasternal intercostal plane blocks in cardiac surgery

37

Why this topic is important

Postoperative pain management in cardiac surgery, particularly following midline sternotomy, is crucial for optimizing recovery and minimizing complications. Sternotomy is associated with severe acute pain, which can lead to respiratory compromise, delayed mobilization, and chronic postsurgical pain if inadequately controlled. Opioids, the mainstay for postoperative pain relief, are limited by adverse effects, including respiratory depression, nausea, constipation, and the risk of dependency.

Traditional regional anesthesia options, such as thoracic epidural and paravertebral blocks, offer effective pain relief but carry risks of complications like epidural hematomas, particularly in anticoagulated patients. Nonsteroidal anti-inflammatory drugs and COX-2 inhibitors are associated with myocardial ischemia and kidney injury, further narrowing the analgesic options.

Superficial parasternal intercostal plane blocks, targeting the anterior cutaneous branches of the thoracic intercostal nerves (fig-1), are emerging as a safe, effective alternative. This technique offers targeted analgesia while avoiding deeper structures, reducing the risk of pleural or vascular injury.

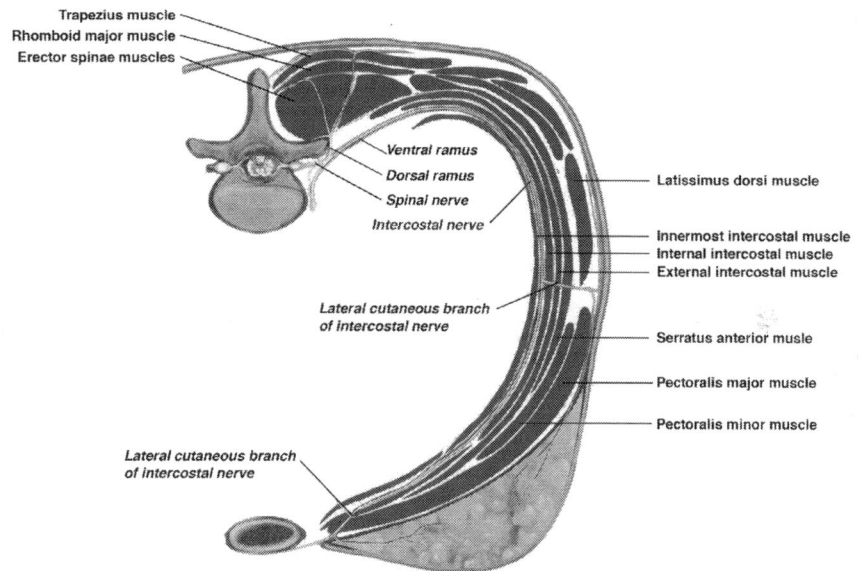

Fig-1. Anatomy of the thoracic spinal and intercostal nerves.
Image taken from NYSORA LMS. https://nysoralms.com/

This update evaluates findings from a systematic review and meta-analysis of randomized controlled trials (RCTs) exploring the role of superficial parasternal intercostal plane blocks in cardiac surgery pain management[1].

Objectives of this update

- Explain the technique and rationale for superficial parasternal intercostal plane blocks.

- Summarize the evidence of their effectiveness in reducing opioid consumption and pain scores.

- Discuss their safety profile and integration into enhanced recovery protocols.

What is new

A systematic review and meta-analysis[1] of 11 RCTs involving 756 patients undergoing sternotomy for cardiac surgery assessed the efficacy and safety of superficial parasternal intercostal plane blocks.

Key findings:

- Reduction in opioid consumption at 24 hours postoperatively by 7.2 mg intravenous (IV) morphine equivalents compared to controls.

- Significant improvements in pain scores up to 24 hours postoperatively.

- Associated reductions in intubation duration and intensive care unit (ICU) length of stay.

- No reported complications among the 196 blocks analyzed.

Detailed findings

Technique overview

The superficial parasternal intercostal plane block involves ultrasound-guided injection of local anesthetic between the internal intercostal and pectoralis major muscles, 2-3 cm lateral to the sternum. This targets the anterior cutaneous branches of the intercostal nerves, which innervate the sternum and anterior chest wall.

Advantages include:

- Safety: Avoids pleural or internal mammary artery injury.

- Ease of performance: Suitable for supine patients, allowing placement intraoperatively or postoperatively.

- Accessibility: Less technically demanding than epidural or paravertebral blocks.

Primary outcomes

1. Opioid consumption:

   - Five trials reported a reduction in opioid consumption at 24 hours by 7.2 mg IV morphine equivalents (moderate-certainty evidence).

   - High heterogeneity was noted, possibly due to variations in block timing and local anesthetic volume.

2. Pain scores:

   - Significant reductions in pain scores were observed at 12, 24, and 48 hours postoperatively.

   - At 24 hours, pain scores were reduced by 1.5 points on a 10-point scale (low-certainty evidence).

Secondary outcomes

1. Intubation time:

   - A reduction of 113 minutes (very low-certainty evidence) in intubation duration was reported in patients receiving the block.

2. ICU length of stay:

   - A reduction of 8.5 hours (moderate-certainty evidence) was observed.

3. Safety:

   - No complications (e.g., pneumothorax, internal mammary artery injury, or local anesthetic toxicity) were reported across five studies analyzing 196 blocks.

Implications for practice

Benefits of superficial parasternal intercostal plane blocks

- Improved pain control: Effective for managing sternotomy pain, with clinically significant reductions in pain scores.

- Opioid-sparing: Reduces the need for systemic opioids, minimizing associated side effects.

- Feasibility: Can be performed intraoperatively or postoperatively without disrupting workflow.

Integration into Enhanced Recovery After Surgery (ERAS) protocols

1. Patient selection:

    ◦ Ideal for patients at risk of opioid-related complications or those contraindicated for epidural analgesia.

2. Technique timing:

    ◦ Can be administered pre- or post-surgery, with similar analgesic outcomes.

Key takeaways

☑ Superficial parasternal intercostal plane blocks provide effective pain relief and reduce opioid consumption after cardiac surgery.

☑ The technique is safe and integrates well into ERAS protocols, offering an alternative to deeper regional blocks.

☑ Further research is needed to standardize practice and optimize outcomes.

Challenges and limitations

1. Heterogeneity in practice:

    ◦ Variability in local anesthetic type, volume, and adjuncts across studies limits generalizability.

2. Outcome measurement:

    ◦ High statistical heterogeneity in pain and opioid consumption outcomes.

3. Sample size:

    ◦ The absence of reported complications is reassuring but may reflect underpowered safety analyses.

Additional recommended reading

1. Cameron MJ, Long J, Kardash K, et al. Superficial parasternal intercostal plane blocks in cardiac surgery: A systematic review and meta-analysis. *Can J Anesth.* 2024;71:883-895.

2. Mittnacht AJ, Shariat A, Weiner MM, et al. Regional techniques for cardiac and cardiac-related procedures. J *Cardiothorac Vasc Anesth.* 2019;33:532-546.

3. Kelava M, Alfirevic A, Bustamante S, et al. Regional anesthesia in cardiac surgery: An overview of fascial plane chest wall blocks. *Anesth Analg.* 2020;131:127-135.

QLB or transversus abdominis plane block for pain control after nephrectomy

38

Why this topic is important

Effective postoperative pain management remains critical for recovery following nephrectomy, a procedure commonly associated with significant postoperative discomfort. Inadequate pain control can delay mobility, prolong hospital stays, and increase the likelihood of chronic pain development. Traditional analgesic approaches, including opioids and neuraxial techniques, are associated with side effects such as sedation, gastrointestinal dysfunction, and risks of hematoma or infection.

Emerging interfascial plane blocks, specifically the transversus abdominis plane block (TAPB) and quadratus lumborum block (QLB), provide localized analgesia that reduces reliance on systemic medications (fig-1). A recent systematic review and network meta-analysis by Gao et al. compares these two regional anesthesia techniques in nephrectomy patients, highlighting their efficacy in opioid reduction, pain relief, and recovery enhancement.

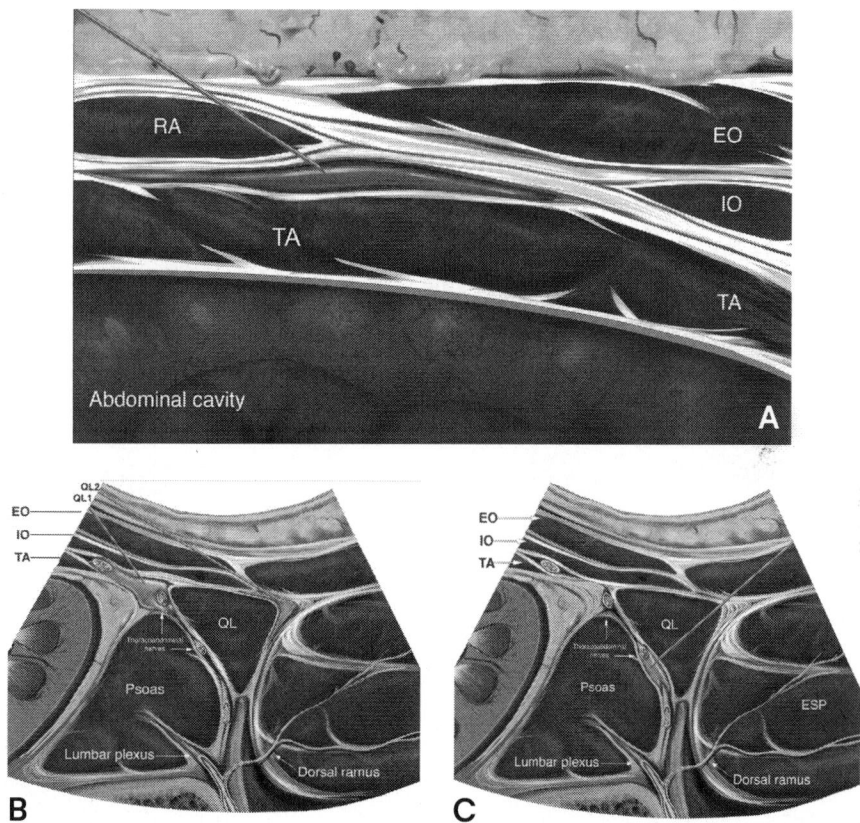

Fig-1A. Reverse ultrasound anatomy of the subcostal TAP block. Needle insertion in-plane from medial to lateral with local anesthetic spread (blue) between transversus abdominis (TA) and rectus abdominis (RA) muscles. EO, external oblique; IO, internal oblique. Fig-1B. Reverse ultrasound anatomy with needle insertion points for QL1 and QL2 blocks. Ideal local anesthetic spread (blue area) for QL1 block - lateral to the QL muscle, and for QL2 block - posterior to the QL muscle. EO, external oblique; IO, internal oblique; TA, transversus abdominis; QL, quadratus lumborum; ESP, erector spinae muscles. Fig-1C. Reverse ultrasound anatomy with needle insertion in-plane for a QL3 block. Ideal local anesthetic distribution (blue) on the anterior aspect of the QL muscle. EO, external oblique; IO, internal oblique; TA, transversus abdominis; QL, quadratus lumborum; ESP, erector spinae muscles. Image taken from NYSORA LMS. https://nysoralms.com/

Objectives of this update

- To compare the analgesic efficacy of TAPB and QLB in patients undergoing nephrectomy.

- To evaluate their impact on opioid consumption, postoperative nausea and vomiting (PONV), pain scores, and hospital length of stay (LOS).

- To guide clinical practice in selecting optimal regional techniques for multimodal pain management.

What is new

The review of Gao et al. 2024 synthesizes findings from 14 studies involving 883 patients, providing the first direct comparison of TAPB and QLB across laparoscopic, open, and robot-assisted nephrectomies. It establishes QLB as the superior technique for reducing opioid use and LOS while highlighting equivalent efficacy for pain intensity and PONV reduction.

Study findings

Methodology

- Design: Systematic review and network meta-analysis.

- Population: 883 patients across 14 studies; 207 received QLB, 245 received TAPB, and 431 received no block or placebo.

- Outcomes: 24-hour opioid consumption (primary), PONV, pain scores, rescue analgesia, and LOS.

Key results

1. Opioid consumption

   - QLB vs. control: QLB significantly reduced 24-hour morphine-equivalent consumption (mean difference: -18.16 mg).

   - TAPB vs. control: No significant reduction (mean difference: -8.34 mg).

   - Network meta-analysis: QLB ranked as the most effective intervention for opioid reduction.

2. Pain scores

   - QLB and TAPB reduced postoperative pain scores at various time points compared to control, but differences between the two blocks were not statistically significant.

3. Rescue analgesia

   - QLB significantly delayed the time it took to rescue analgesia (mean difference: 165 minutes), whereas TAPB had no significant effect.

   - The incidence of rescue analgesia was lower in the QLB group than in the control group.

4. Postoperative nausea and vomiting

   - QLB and TAPB effectively reduced PONV compared to control, with QLB exhibiting slightly better odds ratios.

5. Length of hospital stay

   - QLB significantly reduced LOS.

   - TAPB did not reduce LOS compared to the control.

Clinical implications

QLB is the preferred option for nephrectomy

QLB demonstrated superior efficacy in reducing opioid use, prolonging time to rescue analgesia, and shortening LOS compared to TAPB. These findings make it the preferred choice for multimodal pain management in nephrectomy patients.

Comparable PONV and pain intensity reduction

Both blocks effectively alleviated PONV and postoperative pain scores, supporting their role in enhancing recovery protocols.

Optimizing multimodal strategies

While QLB provides a significant opioid-sparing effect, incorporating it into multimodal analgesia protocols can further enhance outcomes. The lack of impact on LOS with TAPB suggests it may serve as an adjunct rather than a primary analgesic approach.

Limitations

- High heterogeneity in QLB approaches (anterior, posterior, lateral) and variable block execution techniques.

- Limited subgroup analysis on different nephrectomy types and anesthesia methods.

- Inconsistent reporting of pain scores and opioid metrics across studies.

Key takeaways

☑ QLB outperformed TAPB in reducing opioid consumption, prolonging analgesic effects, and shortening hospital stays after nephrectomy.

☑ Both blocks effectively reduced PONV and pain scores, supporting their role in multimodal analgesia.

☑ Incorporating QLB into ERAS protocols could improve recovery outcomes and minimize opioid reliance.

☑ Further research is needed to refine block techniques and optimize patient selection.

Additional recommended reading

1. Gao T, Wang Y, Zheng Y, et al. Quadratus lumborum block vs. transversus abdominis plane block for postoperative pain control in patients with nephrectomy: A systematic review and network meta-analysis. *J Clin Anesth.* 2024;95:111453. doi:10.1016/j.jclinane.2024.111453.

2. El-Boghdadly K, Desai N, Halpern S, et al. Quadratus lumborum block vs. transversus abdominis plane block for cesarean delivery: A systematic review and network meta-analysis. *Anaesthesia.* 2021;76(3):393-403.

3. Korgvee A, Veskimae E, Huhtala H, et al. Posterior quadratus lumborum block versus epidural analgesia for postoperative pain management after open radical cystectomy: A randomized clinical trial. *Acta Anaesthesiol Scand.* 2023;67(3):347-55.

Serratus plane block or standard care for pain after endoscopic aortic valve replacement

39

Why this topic is important

Endoscopic aortic valve replacement (TEAVR) is an innovative, minimally invasive cardiac surgery technique that eliminates the need for sternotomy, reducing surgical trauma and promoting faster recovery. Despite these advances, postoperative pain management remains a challenge, with opioids often forming the cornerstone of analgesic regimens. Opioids, however, are associated with significant side effects, including respiratory depression, nausea, and the risk of long-term dependency.

The ultrasound-guided serratus anterior plane block (SAPB) has shown promise in reducing opioid requirements in thoracic and chest wall surgeries (fig-1). Still, its role in cardiac surgery has yet to be explored. A recent study by Vandenbrande et al.[1] evaluates the efficacy of SAPB compared to standard care for pain management after TEAVR, potentially supporting its integration into enhanced recovery after cardiac surgery (ERACS) protocols.

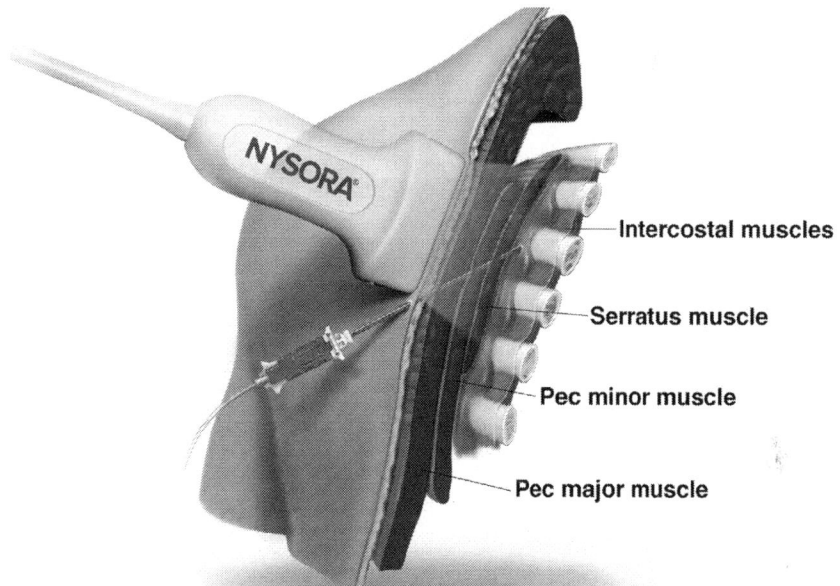

Fig-1. Transducer position and needle insertion in-plane with local anesthetic spread underneath the serratus anterior muscle for a serratus anterior plane block.
Image taken from NYSORA LMS. https://nysoralms.com/

Objectives of this update

- To assess the efficacy of SAPB in reducing opioid consumption during the first 24 hours postoperatively.

- To evaluate its impact on pain intensity, opioid-free outcomes, and patient satisfaction.

- To determine the feasibility of incorporating SAPB into postoperative pain management protocols for TEAVR.

What is new

This is the first double-blind, randomized controlled trial to demonstrate that a single-injection SAPB significantly reduces opioid requirements and pain scores after TEAVR, outperforming standard care analgesia.

Study findings

Study design and population

- Design: Double-blind, single-center, prospective, randomized controlled trial.

- Participants: 75 adult patients undergoing TEAVR, randomized 1:1 into two groups:

  ◦ SAPB group: Received a combined deep and superficial SAPB with 40 mL of 0.25% bupivacaine upon intensive care unit (ICU) admission, alongside standard multimodal analgesia.

  ◦ Control group: Received standard multimodal analgesia without SAPB.

- Exclusion criteria: Chronic pain, opioid use, morbid obesity, low body weight, or prior chest trauma/surgery.

Results

1. Opioid consumption

   ◦ Median 24-hour opioid use was significantly lower in the SAPB group (9 morphine milligram equivalents [MME]) compared to the control group (15 MME).

   ◦ The SAPB group consistently required fewer opioids during all measured intervals.

2. Pain intensity

   ◦ At multiple time points, the SAPB group's pain scores (Numeric Rating Scale [NRS]) at rest were significantly reduced.

3. Opioid-free patients and adverse events

   ◦ Two patients in the SAPB group were opioid-free at 24 hours, compared to none in the control group.

   ◦ No significant differences in adverse events, including nausea, vomiting, or constipation, were observed between groups.

4. Secondary outcomes

   ◦ Quality of recovery and patient satisfaction were higher in the SAPB group but did not reach statistical significance.

   ◦ No differences in ICU or hospital length of stay were identified.

Clinical implications

Benefits of SAPB in TEAVR

- Opioid-sparing effect: SAPB reduced opioid use by over 25%, meeting the study's primary endpoint and addressing a critical aspect of postoperative care in minimizing opioid-related risks.

- Enhanced pain control: Lower pain scores at rest indicate that SAPB improves patient comfort during critical early recovery.

- Feasibility: SAPB is a safe, ultrasound-guided technique that can be integrated into ERACS protocols without disrupting clinical workflows.

Considerations for practice

- SAPB offers an effective alternative to solely opioid-based regimens, particularly for patients with higher risks of opioid-related complications.

- Its use may be particularly beneficial in centers prioritizing minimally invasive techniques and enhanced recovery pathways.

Limitations and future directions

Study limitations

- The single-center design may limit generalizability to other institutions or surgical populations.
- Sample size and limited follow-up preclude conclusions on long-term opioid use and recovery outcomes.

Future research

- Larger multicenter trials to confirm findings and explore outcomes in diverse patient populations.
- Comparisons of SAPB with other regional anesthesia techniques in cardiac and thoracic surgeries.
- Investigations into the optimal timing, volume, and drug combinations for SAPB.

Key takeaways

☑ SAPB significantly reduces opioid use and pain scores within the first 24 hours after TEAVR compared to standard care.

☑ The block offers a safe, effective addition to multimodal analgesia in ERACS protocols.

☑ SAPB's integration into routine care for minimally invasive cardiac surgeries warrants further exploration.

Additional recommended reading

1. Vandenbrande J, Jamaer B, Stessel B, et al. Serratus plane block versus standard of care for pain control after totally endoscopic aortic valve replacement: A double-blind, randomized controlled, superiority trial. *Reg Anesth Pain Med.* 2024;49:429-435.

2. Blanco R, Parras T, McDonnell JG, et al. Serratus plane block: A novel ultrasound-guided thoracic wall nerve block. *Anaesthesia.* 2013;68:1107-13.

3. Jack JM, McLellan E, Versyck B, et al. The role of serratus anterior plane and pectoral nerves blocks in cardiac surgery, thoracic surgery, and trauma: A qualitative systematic review. *Anaesthesia.* 2020;75:1372-85.

Innovations in block techniques and pain management

Intrathecal bupivacaine or mepivacaine for same-day discharge total joint arthroplasty

40

Why this topic is important

The shift toward same-day discharge total joint arthroplasty (TJA), driven by bundled payment models and the demands of surgical efficiency, has increased the importance of optimizing anesthetic protocols. Intrathecal (IT) anesthesia is commonly used for TJA, offering reliable sensory and motor blockade while avoiding the risks of general anesthesia. However, the choice of local anesthetic plays a critical role in determining the duration of motor block, time to mobilization, and discharge readiness.

Hyperbaric bupivacaine is a standard IT agent due to its effective and predictable blockade, but its prolonged duration can delay discharge. Isobaric mepivacaine, with a shorter and more predictable resolution of motor and sensory blockade, may be better suited for outpatient TJAs. A recent study by Coleman et al. 2024 evaluates the impact of transitioning from IT bupivacaine to IT mepivacaine in a large academic medical center performing same-day discharge TJA.

Objectives of this update

- To compare postoperative recovery times and outcomes between IT bupivacaine and IT mepivacaine.

- To assess the effect of mepivacaine on post-anesthesia care unit (PACU) discharge readiness and opioid consumption.

- To identify potential trade-offs between faster recovery and increased pain management needs.

What is new

The study of Coleman et al. 2024 is one of the first to evaluate IT mepivacaine for TJA in a complex academic setting. It highlights faster PACU discharge times with mepivacaine but also underscores the need for balancing increased opioid use and higher postoperative pain scores.

Study findings

Methodology

- Design: Retrospective quality improvement study involving 96 patients undergoing same-day discharge TJA (hip or knee arthroplasty).

- Groups:

  ○ Bupivacaine group: 44 patients received 1.2-1.4 mL hyperbaric bupivacaine 0.75%.

  ○ Mepivacaine group: 48 patients received 2.5-3 mL isobaric mepivacaine 1.5%.

- Outcomes: PACU discharge time, perioperative opioid consumption, PACU pain scores, and conversion rates to general anesthesia or overnight admission.

Results

1. PACU discharge times

   ∘ The median discharge time was significantly shorter in the mepivacaine group (4.03 hours) than in the bupivacaine group (5.33 hours).

2. Pain scores

   ∘ The mepivacaine group had higher pain scores in PACU (arrival pain score: 3.08 vs. 0.87; maximum pain score: 6.29 vs. 3.41).

3. Opioid consumption

   ∘ Perioperative opioid consumption was significantly higher in the mepivacaine group (22.5 mg vs. 11.4 mg).

4. Complications and admissions

   ∘ No significant differences in conversion to general anesthesia or overnight admission were observed between groups.

Clinical implications

Benefits of faster recovery with mepivacaine

The shorter PACU discharge times observed with mepivacaine can improve bed turnover and reduce resource strain, especially in high-demand settings. This is particularly relevant for academic medical centers dealing with patient surges or bed shortages.

Managing pain and opioid use

The trade-off for faster block resolution with mepivacaine is higher early postoperative pain and increased opioid requirements. Effective pain management strategies, such as multimodal analgesia, are critical when using mepivacaine to ensure patient comfort and minimize opioid-related side effects.

Patient selection

Mepivacaine may be best suited for patients undergoing shorter procedures or those with a strong support system for managing postoperative pain at home. Its rapid block resolution aligns with the goals of outpatient TJA, but careful patient education and discharge planning are essential.

Advantages and disadvantages of intrathecal mepivacaine vs. bupivacaine for same-day discharge TJA	
Advantages	**Disadvantages**
Faster PACU discharge times: Median discharge time reduced to 4.03 hours with mepivacaine compared to 5.33 hours with bupivacaine	**Higher postoperative pain scores:** Increased PACU pain scores, with a maximum score of 6.29 vs. 3.41 for bupivacaine.
More predictable block resolution: Mepivacaine allows earlier ambulation and better aligns with outpatient surgery protocols.	**Increased opioid consumption:** Mean perioperative opioid use was 22.5 mg with mepivacaine compared to 11.4 mg with bupivacaine.
Avoidance of overnight admission: Both anesthetics showed similar low rates of unplanned admissions (2.1% for mepivacaine vs. 2.3% for bupivacaine).	**Shorter sensory and motor block duration:** May necessitate more aggressive early postoperative analgesia.
Efficient use of hospital resources: Reduced PACU length of stay enhances bed turnover and decreases strain on resources	**Potential patient discomfort:** Higher pain scores on PACU arrival may require more intensive management.

Limitations and future directions

Study limitations

- Retrospective design: Potential for selection bias and uncontrolled confounders.

- Single-surgeon cohort: Results may not generalize to other settings or surgical teams.

- Limited pain management data: The study did not assess post-discharge opioid use or patient-reported pain scores at home.

Recommendations for future research

- Investigate long-term outcomes, including opioid use and patient satisfaction, with IT mepivacaine versus bupivacaine.

- Explore the use of adjuncts like clonidine or dexamethasone to enhance analgesia without prolonging block duration.

- Conduct prospective trials to confirm findings and refine patient selection criteria.

Key takeaways

- ☑ Intrathecal mepivacaine significantly reduces PACU discharge times compared to bupivacaine, supporting its use in same-day discharge TJA.

- ☑ The trade-off for faster recovery is higher PACU pain scores and increased perioperative opioid consumption.

- ☑ Effective multimodal analgesia and discharge planning are essential to maximize the benefits of mepivacaine in outpatient TJA.

- ☑ Further research is needed to validate findings and optimize anesthetic protocols for same-day discharge surgeries.

Additional recommended reading

1. Coleman PW, Underriner TC, Kennerley VM, Marshall KD. Transitioning from intrathecal bupivacaine to mepivacaine for same-day discharge total joint arthroplasty: A quality improvement study. *Reg Anesth Pain Med*. 2024;49:254-259.

2. Schwenk ES, Kasper VP, Smoker JD, et al. Mepivacaine versus bupivacaine spinal anesthesia for early postoperative ambulation. *Anesthesiology*. 2020;133:801-11.

3. Calkins TE, McClatchy SG, Rider CM, et al. Mepivacaine vs bupivacaine spinal anesthesia in total hip arthroplasty at an ambulatory surgery center. *J Arthroplasty*. 2021;36:3676-80.

Bilateral ultrasound-guided maxillary and mandibular nerve blocks in orthognathic surgery

41

Why this topic is important

Double-jaw orthognathic surgery, a procedure used to correct maxillofacial abnormalities, is associated with significant postoperative pain. Effective pain management in these cases often requires opioids, leading to potential side effects such as nausea, sedation, and dependency. Regional anesthesia (RA), particularly maxillary (V2) and mandibular (V3) nerve blocks (fig-1) has emerged as a promising strategy to reduce opioid use and enhance recovery outcomes.

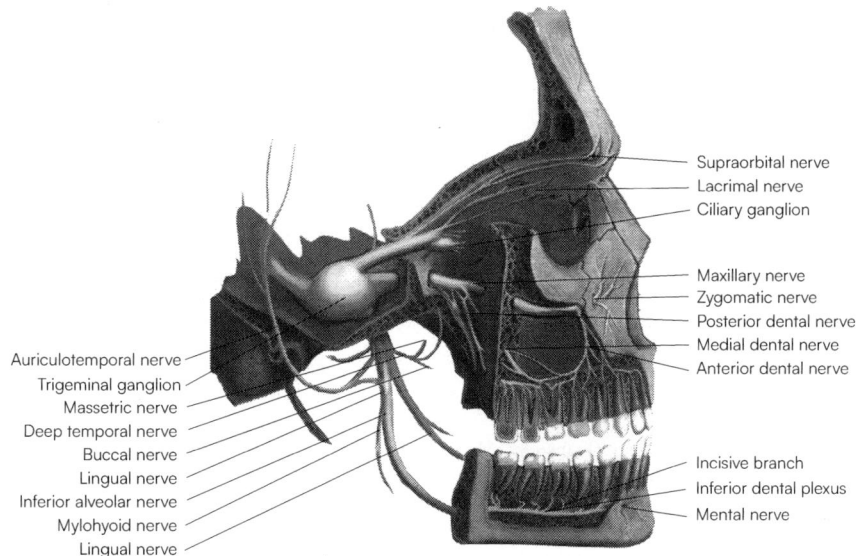

Fig-1. Anatomy of the trigeminal nerve. The sensory root of the trigeminal nerve gives rise to the ophthalmic division, maxillary division, and mandibular division.
Image taken from NYSORA LMS. https://nysoralms.com/

The study by Esquerré et al. 2024 investigates the efficacy of bilateral ultrasound-guided maxillary and mandibular nerve blocks in minimizing opioid consumption and improving postoperative pain management, offering an alternative to traditional approaches that rely heavily on systemic analgesia.

Objectives of this update

- To assess the impact of bilateral V2 and V3 nerve blocks on postoperative opioid consumption in double-jaw surgery.

- To compare the analgesic efficacy of ultrasound-guided nerve blocks versus local infiltration of anesthetics.

- To evaluate the safety and feasibility of ultrasound-guided regional anesthesia in maxillofacial surgery.

What is new

This randomized controlled trial by Esquerré et al. 2024 demonstrates that ultrasound-guided V2 and V3 nerve blocks reduce postoperative morphine consumption by 50% within the first 24 hours compared to intraoral infiltration. It establishes a clinically significant role for regional anesthesia in maxillofacial surgery.

Study findings

Methodology

- Design: Single-blind randomized controlled trial conducted at a French university hospital from May 2022 to July 2023.

- Participants: 50 patients aged 15-45 undergoing elective double-jaw orthognathic surgery.

- Interventions:

  ○ Regional Anesthesia (RA) group: Bilateral ultrasound-guided V2 and V3 nerve blocks using 5 mL of 4.75 mg/mL ropivacaine per block.

  ○ Infiltration group: Intraoral infiltration using 10 mg/mL lidocaine with epinephrine.

- Primary outcome: Cumulative oral morphine equivalent (OME) consumption at postoperative day 1 (POD1).

- Secondary outcomes: OME at 48 hours, pain scores, opioid-related side effects, and correlation between preoperative anxiety and postoperative pain.

Key results

1. Primary outcome: OME at 24 hours

   ○ Patients in the RA group had significantly lower cumulative oral morphine equivalent (OME) consumption at postoperative day 1 (25.5 ± 19.8 mg) compared to those in the infiltration group (45.7 ± 37.6 mg).

   ○ This represents a 50% reduction in opioid use in the first 24 hours, indicating that bilateral V2 and V3 nerve blocks provide substantial opioid-sparing benefits during the critical early postoperative period.

   ○ The difference in OME highlights the effectiveness of RA in minimizing reliance on systemic analgesia, which is a key goal in optimizing postoperative recovery.

2. Secondary outcomes

   ○ OME at 48 hours: The RA group demonstrated lower opioid consumption at 48 hours (35.8 ± 30.2 mg) than the infiltration group (64.5 ± 60.0 mg).

   ○ Pain scores: No significant difference in maximum numerical rating scale (NRS) pain scores between groups.

   ○ Preoperative anxiety: Higher preoperative anxiety levels were associated with greater opioid use and worse pain scores on postoperative day 2

3. Safety and feasibility

   ○ A single minor complication (vascular puncture during the V3 nerve block) was observed in the RA group, with no significant clinical consequences.

   ○ No reported cases of systemic toxicity, infection, or major adverse events confirmed the safety of ultrasound-guided regional anesthesia in this surgical population.

Clinical implications

Pain relief and opioid-sparing benefits

The study underscores the effectiveness of bilateral V2 and V3 nerve blocks in reducing opioid requirements, potentially mitigating the side effects and risks of systemic analgesia. This reduction can significantly benefit patients by minimizing opioid-related complications like postoperative nausea and dependency.

Implementation in practice

- Technique feasibility: Ultrasound guidance enhances safety and precision, particularly in complex anatomical areas.

- Patient selection: Ideal for patients undergoing procedures with high pain burdens, such as double-jaw surgery, or those at risk of opioid-related adverse events.

Limitations of RA in maxillofacial surgery

- While RA significantly reduced opioid use, pain scores between groups were comparable. This could be attributed to the multimodal analgesia protocol and limitations in addressing residual pain from areas not covered by the nerve block (e.g., V1 territory).

Limitations

- Single-blind design: Blinding was limited to postoperative caregivers; the operating team was aware of group assignments.

- Agent variability: Different local anesthetics were used for RA and infiltration groups, potentially influencing results.

- Short follow-up duration: Long-term outcomes, including chronic pain prevention, were not assessed.

Key takeaways

☑ Bilateral ultrasound-guided V2 and V3 nerve blocks reduce postoperative opioid consumption by 50% in double-jaw orthognathic surgery.

☑ Pain scores were similar between groups, emphasizing the importance of multimodal analgesia.

☑ Preoperative anxiety correlates with higher pain and opioid use, highlighting the need for holistic perioperative care.

☑ Ultrasound-guided RA is safe, feasible, and effective, representing a valuable addition to perioperative pain management strategies in maxillofacial surgery.

Additional recommended reading

1. Esquerré T, Mure M, Minville V, et al. Bilateral ultrasound-guided maxillary and mandibular combined nerves block reduces morphine consumption after double-jaw orthognathic surgery: A randomized controlled trial. *Reg Anesth Pain Med.* 2024;49:1-6.

2. Molins G, Valls-Ontañón A, De Nadal M, et al. Ultrasound-guided suprazygomatic maxillary nerve block is effective in reducing postoperative opioid use following bimaxillary osteotomy. *J Oral Maxillofac Surg.* 2024;82:412-21.

3. Chiono J, Raux O, Bringuier S, et al. Bilateral suprazygomatic maxillary nerve block for cleft palate repair in children: A prospective, randomized, double-blind study versus placebo. *Anesthesiology.* 2014;120:1362-9.

Liposomal bupivacaine in supraclavicular brachial plexus blocks

42

Why this topic is important

The supraclavicular brachial plexus block (fig-1) is a widely used technique for regional anesthesia in upper extremity surgeries, such as distal radial fracture fixation. While effective, the duration of single-injection blocks is often limited, with patients experiencing rebound pain as the block wears off. Liposomal bupivacaine, a sustained-release formulation, has shown promise in extending the duration of analgesia in other types of nerve blocks. However, its role in the supraclavicular block still needs to be explored.

Chan et al. 2024 investigate whether adding liposomal bupivacaine to standard bupivacaine in supraclavicular brachial plexus blocks improves pain control and enhances patient outcomes. The findings contribute to optimizing regional anesthesia strategies for postoperative pain management.

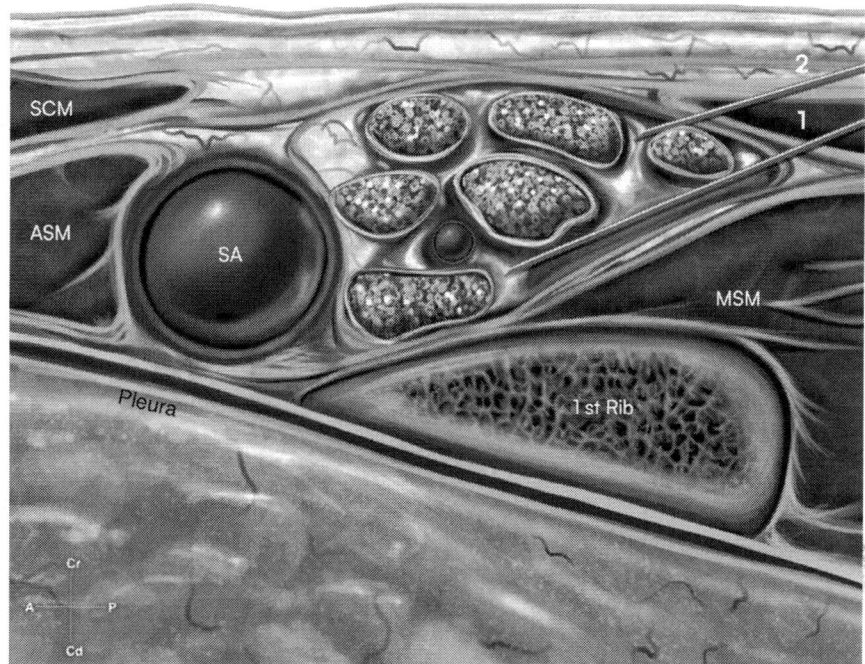

Fig-1. Supraclavicular brachial plexus block; Reverse ultrasound anatomy with needle insertion in-plane. SA, subclavian artery; MSM, middle scalene muscle; SCM, sternocleidomastoid muscle; ASM, anterior scalene muscle. Image taken from NYSORA LMS. https://nysoralms.com/

Objectives of this update

- To evaluate the efficacy of liposomal bupivacaine in extending postoperative analgesia in supraclavicular blocks.

- To compare pain control and functional recovery between liposomal bupivacaine and standard bupivacaine groups.

- To explore potential implications for clinical practice in regional anesthesia.

What is new

This randomized controlled trial by Chan et al. 2024 is the first to assess the addition of liposomal bupivacaine in supraclavicular brachial plexus blocks. The study reveals significant improvements in early postoperative pain control, particularly during the first 48 hours, when liposomal bupivacaine is combined with standard bupivacaine.

Study findings

Methodology

- Design: A double-blind, randomized controlled trial with 80 patients undergoing distal radial fracture fixation.

- Interventions:

  ○ Liposomal group: 10 mL of 0.5% plain bupivacaine immediately followed by 10 mL of 1.33% liposomal bupivacaine.

  ○ Standard group: 20 mL of 0.5% plain bupivacaine.

- Primary outcome: Weighted area under the curve (AUC) of pain scores at rest over the first 48 hours.

- Secondary outcomes: Pain with movement, opioid consumption, sleep quality, and functional recovery scores.

Results

1. Pain control

   ○ Weighted AUC pain score at rest in the first 48 hours was significantly lower in the liposomal group (0.6 vs. 1.4).

   ○ Weighted AUC pain scores with movement in the first 48 hours were also lower in the liposomal group (2.3 vs 3.7).

   ○ By postoperative day 2, differences in pain scores were no longer significant.

2. Opioid consumption and sleep quality

   ○ No significant differences were observed in total oxycodone consumption or sleep disturbance scores between groups.

3. Functional recovery

   ○ No meaningful differences in sensory or motor function, grip strength, or longer-term outcomes (e.g., QuickDASH and SF-12v2 scores) were found between groups.

4. Safety

   ○ There were no reports of nerve block-related adverse effects, including respiratory compromise or local anesthetic toxicity.

Clinical implications

Enhanced early pain control

The addition of liposomal bupivacaine provided superior pain relief during the first 48 hours after surgery, addressing the critical period of acute postoperative pain. However, the benefit was most pronounced on postoperative day 1, with diminishing effects afterward.

Considerations for clinical practice

- Patient selection: Liposomal bupivacaine may be particularly valuable for patients at high risk of significant rebound pain or those undergoing surgeries with high postoperative pain burdens.

- Cost and availability: Given its higher cost, judicious use in select patient populations is warranted until broader evidence supports routine use.

- Feasibility: The combined injection with plain bupivacaine ensures rapid onset for surgical anesthesia, making it practical for use in clinical settings.

Long-term outcomes

The absence of significant differences in longer-term functional outcomes suggests that liposomal bupivacaine's primary advantage lies in its early postoperative analgesic benefits rather than sustained recovery advantages.

Limitations and future directions

Study limitations

- Short duration of effect: The analgesic benefits of liposomal bupivacaine were limited to the early postoperative period.

- Lack of functional primary outcomes: Pain scores at rest may not fully capture the functional implications of improved analgesia.

- Restricted generalizability: Findings are specific to distal radial fracture surgeries and may not apply to other upper extremity procedures.

Recommendations for future research

- Investigate the role of liposomal bupivacaine in ambulatory surgery and high-risk patient populations.

- Explore combinations with adjuvants, such as dexamethasone, to enhance its duration of effect.

- Conduct cost-effectiveness analyses to assess the value of routine use in regional anesthesia.

Key takeaways

☑ Adding liposomal bupivacaine to supraclavicular blocks significantly improves pain control during the first 48 hours post-surgery, especially on day 1.

☑ No significant reductions in opioid use or long-term functional recovery were observed, suggesting limited overall impact on extended outcomes.

☑ Liposomal bupivacaine may be best suited for patients at risk of severe rebound pain or for surgeries associated with high acute pain levels.

☑ Further studies are needed to confirm its utility across diverse surgical and patient populations.

Additional recommended reading

1. Chan TCW, Wong JSH, Wang F, et al. Addition of liposomal bupivacaine to standard bupivacaine versus standard bupivacaine alone in the supraclavicular brachial plexus block: A randomized controlled trial. *Anesthesiology*. 2024;141(4):732-744.

2. Ilfeld BM, Eisenach JC, Gabriel RA. Clinical effectiveness of liposomal bupivacaine in peripheral nerve blocks. *Anesthesiology*. 2021;134:283-344.

3. Joshi G, Gandhi K, Shah N, Gadsden J, Corman SL. Peripheral nerve blocks in the management of postoperative pain: challenges and opportunities. *J Clin Anesth*. 2016 Dec;35:524-529.

Liposomal bupivacaine in sciatic nerve blocks after bunionectomy

43

Why this topic is important

Foot and ankle surgeries, such as bunionectomy, are associated with moderate-to-severe postoperative pain, particularly within the first three days after surgery. Effective pain management strategies are essential to enhance recovery, minimize opioid consumption, and improve patient satisfaction. Traditional approaches, such as single-shot or continuous infusion of bupivacaine hydrochloride (HCl), offer temporary relief but require alternative methods for prolonged analgesia.

Liposomal bupivacaine (LB) provides sustained local anesthetic release, offering potential advantages in peripheral nerve blocks for prolonged postoperative pain control. The phase 3 trial by Schartz et al. 2024 evaluates LB administered via a popliteal sciatic nerve block, comparing it to conventional bupivacaine HCl in bunionectomy patients.

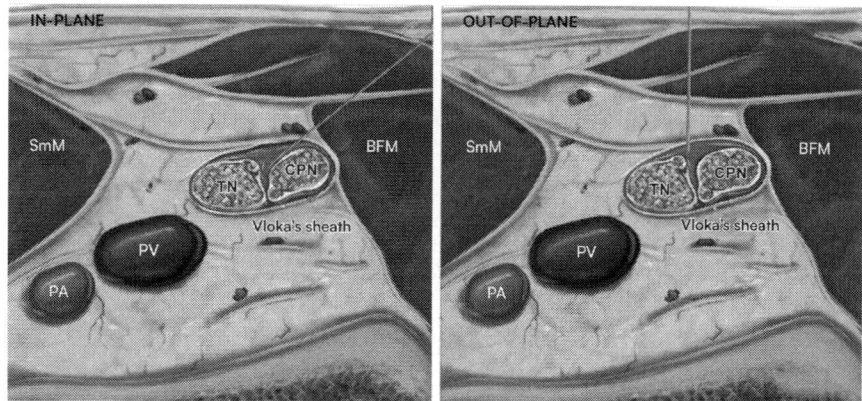

Fig-1. Reverse ultrasound anatomy of a popliteal sciatic nerve block. Local anesthetic spread surrounding the sciatic nerve within the Vloka's sheath using an in-plane (left) or out-of-plane (right) approach. TN, tibial nerve; CPN, common peroneal nerve; PV popliteal vein; PA, popliteal artery; SmM, semimembranosus muscle; BFM, biceps femoris muscle.
Image taken from NYSORA LMS. https://nysoralms.com/

Objectives of this update

- To compare the analgesic efficacy and duration of pain control provided by LB versus bupivacaine HCl.

- To examine opioid consumption and opioid-free rates over a 96-hour postoperative period.

- To evaluate safety and patient satisfaction associated with LB.

What is new

The study of Schwartz et al. 2024 demonstrates that LB significantly reduces pain scores, decreases opioid consumption, and increases opioid-free rates up to 96 hours after surgery compared to bupivacaine HCl.

Study findings

Methodology

- Design: Multicenter, randomized, double-blind, active-controlled trial.

- Participants: 185 adults undergoing elective bunionectomy with ASA classification ≤3.

- Intervention:

  ○ LB 133 mg or 266 mg versus bupivacaine HCl 50 mg, administered via ultrasound-guided popliteal sciatic nerve block.

  ○ All participants received adjunctive analgesics, including IV acetaminophen and a Mayo field block with bupivacaine.

- The primary endpoint is the area under the curve (AUC) of the numerical rating scale (NRS) pain scores over 96 hours.

- Secondary endpoints: Opioid consumption, opioid-free rates, time to first opioid, and participant satisfaction.

Results

1. Pain scores

   ○ LB 133 mg reduced the AUC of NRS pain scores by 44% compared to bupivacaine HCl over 96 hours.

   ○ Pain scores were similar in the first 24 hours but consistently lower in the LB group from 24 to 96 hours.

2. Opioid consumption

   ○ LB 133 mg resulted in a 61% reduction in total opioid use compared to bupivacaine HCl.

   ○ At 96 hours, 24.4% of participants in the LB group were opioid-free, compared to 6.0% in the bupivacaine group.

3. Participant satisfaction

   ○ Both groups reported high satisfaction, indicating effective pain control.

4. Safety

   ○ Adverse event rates were similar between groups, with most events mild to moderate.

   ○ Nausea and dizziness were the most common side effects in both groups.

Clinical implications

Advantages of liposomal bupivacaine

LB provides extended pain relief beyond the active period of bupivacaine HCl, reducing the need for rescue analgesics. This is particularly beneficial for outpatient surgeries like bunionectomy, where patients must self-manage pain at home.

Potential for opioid-free recovery

By increasing opioid-free rates and reducing overall opioid requirements, LB may contribute to addressing the opioid crisis while improving recovery trajectories.

Practical considerations

- LB's extended duration reduces the need for continuous nerve block catheters, minimizing risks such as infection or catheter dislodgment.

- Despite higher costs associated with LB, the reduction in opioid use and hospital resources may justify its integration into multimodal analgesia protocols.

Limitations

- Population specificity: Results may not generalize to other surgical procedures or patient populations.

- Adjunctive analgesics: Using multimodal analgesia in both groups could dilute the apparent benefits of LB.

Key takeaways

☑ Liposomal bupivacaine significantly reduces pain scores and opioid consumption compared to bupivacaine HCl up to 96 hours post-bunionectomy.

☑ The increased proportion of opioid-free participants highlights LB's role in promoting safer postoperative recovery.

☑ LB offers an effective alternative to continuous infusion techniques, with similar safety profiles.

Additional recommended reading

1. Schwartz G, Gadsden JC, Gonzales J, et al. A phase 3 active-controlled trial of liposomal bupivacaine via sciatic nerve block in the popliteal fossa after bunionectomy. *J Clin Anesth.* 2024;94:111402.

2. Joshi GP, Gandhi K, Shah N, et al. Peripheral nerve blocks in the management of postoperative pain: challenges and opportunities. *J Clin Anesth.* 2020;64:109835.

3. Chou LB, Wagner D, Witten DM, et al. Postoperative pain following foot and ankle surgery: a prospective study. *Foot Ankle Int.* 2008;29(11):1063-1068.

Trends in liposomal bupivacaine utilization in lower extremity joint arthroplasty

44

Why this topic is important

Liposomal bupivacaine (LB) was introduced as an extended-release local anesthetic intended to provide prolonged postoperative analgesia for up to 72 hours (fig-1). Its use gained traction in total hip and knee arthroplasty (THA/TKA), procedures associated with significant postoperative pain. LB promised to reduce reliance on additional analgesics, including opioids, while improving patient outcomes.

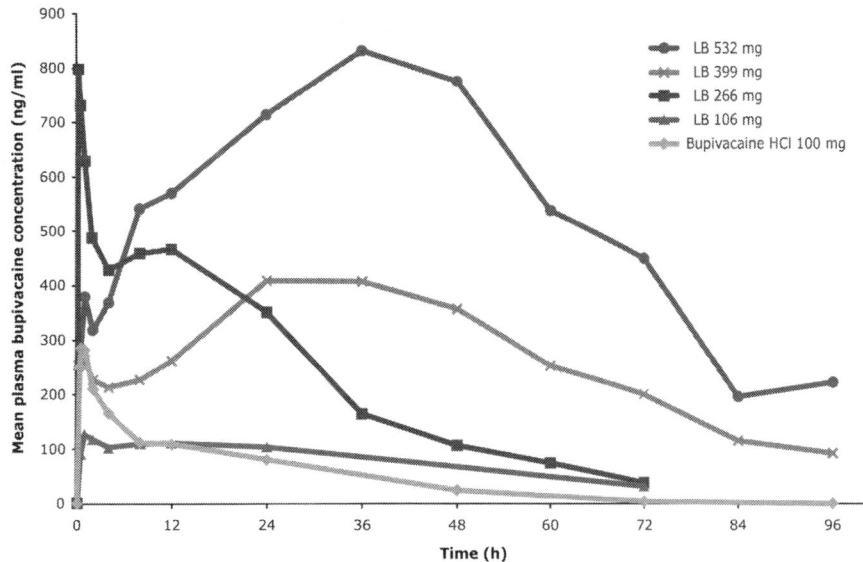

Fig-1. Plasma bupivacaine concentration versus time for liposome bupivacaine 106, 266, 399, and 532 mg, and bupivacaine HCL 100 mg. LB, liposome bupivacaine. Figure adapted from Hu et al. 2013.

However, the high cost of LB, coupled with mixed evidence regarding its efficacy compared to plain bupivacaine, has raised questions about its value. The population-based study by Studner el at. 2024 provides a comprehensive analysis of trends in LB utilization across the United States over 10 years, offering insights into its evolving role in perioperative pain management.

Objectives of this update

- To evaluate temporal trends in the utilization of LB for THA/TKA at the individual and hospital levels.

- To identify factors influencing the initiation and termination of LB use.

- To explore implications for clinical practice, policy, and cost-effectiveness in arthroplasty.

What is new

The study by Stundner et al. 2024 is the first to document a national decline in LB utilization after an initial surge in adoption, highlighting regional and institutional variability in its use and retention.

Study findings

Methodology

- Design: Retrospective observational analysis using the Premier Healthcare Database (2012-2021).

- Participants: 2,541,367 adult patients undergoing elective THA or TKA.

- Exposure: LB use identified via pharmacy billing codes.

- Outcomes: Trends in LB use at the patient and hospital levels, including initiation and termination rates.

Results

1. LB Use at the patient level

   ○ LB utilization increased rapidly from 0.4% in 2012 to a peak of 22.8% in 2015.

   ○ After 2015, LB use declined annually by 1-3%, with only 15.7% of TJA cases utilizing LB by 2021.

   ○ Over the study period, LB was used in 16.6% of TJA cases.

2. LB Use at the hospital level

   ○ Of 1,003 hospitals performing TJA, 59.7% used LB at some point.

   ○ Initiation of LB peaked in 2014 (32.8%) but decreased to just 4.3% in 2021.

   ○ Termination rates rose significantly, reaching 9.9% by 2019.

   ○ Non-teaching hospitals and those in the South and West regions retained LB use longer than teaching or Midwest/Northeast hospitals.

3. Survival analysis

   ○ Kaplan-Meier curves showed a faster decline in LB use among teaching hospitals, likely reflecting quicker adoption of evidence questioning its cost-effectiveness.

   ○ Regional disparities suggest varying responses to clinical and economic pressures.

Clinical implications

Diminishing popularity of LB

The decline in LB use after 2015 coincides with increasing evidence questioning its efficacy. While initial studies suggested modest benefits, subsequent randomized controlled trials (RCTs) and meta-analyses failed to demonstrate clinically meaningful advantages over plain bupivacaine.

Economic considerations

LB's high cost ($365.15 per 20 mL dose) remains a significant barrier. Despite theoretical savings from reduced opioid use and shorter hospital stays, most studies have not shown consistent cost benefits. For many institutions, alternative local anesthetics offer comparable outcomes at a fraction of the price.

Regional and institutional variability

- Non-teaching hospitals and those in the South/West regions were slower in terminating LB use, possibly due to fewer academic affiliations and slower adoption of emerging evidence.

- Teaching hospitals and those in the Northeast/Midwest appear more responsive to literature questioning LB's utility, likely due to a stronger emphasis on evidence-based practice.

Key takeaways

☑ LB use in THA/TKA peaked in 2015 but has steadily declined, with only 15.7% of cases utilizing LB by 2021.

☑ Teaching hospitals and those in the Northeast/Midwest were quicker to discontinue LB, likely reflecting a stronger emphasis on cost-effectiveness and evidence-based practice.

☑ Regional and institutional disparities highlight the need for standardized guidelines on LB's use in arthroplasty.

☑ Further research is necessary to determine whether LB's high cost can be justified in select patient populations or surgical contexts.

Additional recommended reading

1. Stundner O, Hoerner E, Zhong H, et al. Trends of liposomal bupivacaine utilization in major lower extremity total joint arthroplasty in the USA: a population-based study. *Reg Anesth Pain Med.* 2024;49:139-143.

2. Hussain N, Brull R, Sheehy B, et al. Perineural liposomal bupivacaine is not superior to nonliposomal bupivacaine for peripheral nerve block analgesia. *Anesthesiology.* 2021;134:147-64.

3. Dinges HC, Wiesmann T, Otremba B, et al. The analgesic efficacy of liposomal bupivacaine compared with bupivacaine hydrochloride for the prevention of postoperative pain: a systematic review and meta-analysis. *Reg Anesth Pain Med.* 2021;46:490-8.

4. Hu D, Onel E, Singla N, et al. Pharmacokinetic profile of liposome bupivacaine injection following a single administration at the surgical site. *Clin Drug Investig.* 2013;33:109-15.

Parasternal intercostal plane block for analgesia

45

Why this topic is important

Parasternal intercostal plane (PIP) blocks, targeting the anterior cutaneous branches of the T2-T6 intercostal nerves, are increasingly used for effective postoperative analgesia following chest wall and cardiac surgeries, including sternotomies and mastectomies. These blocks are essential in reducing pain and opioid requirements, yet the optimal techniques to maximize their efficacy remain unclear. A recent cadaveric study by Samerchua et al. (2024) evaluates the ideal number and locations of injections for superficial and deep PIP blocks, providing critical insights for improved clinical application and patient outcomes.

Objectives of this update

- To identify the optimal injection sites and techniques for ultrasound-guided superficial and deep PIP blocks.

- To evaluate the dye spread and coverage of intercostal spaces achieved by different techniques.

- To provide anatomical and sonographic insights for safer and more effective PIP block administration.

What is new

This study by Samerchua et al. (2024) introduces a systematic approach to PIP blocks. It demonstrates that multiple injections improve dye spread and coverage and makes specific recommendations for injection points in superficial and deep techniques.

Key findings

Study design and methodology

- Sample: 12 cadavers (24 hemithoraces).

- Techniques tested: Superficial injections at 1-3 sites (second, fourth, fifth intercostal spaces) and deep injections at 1-2 sites (third, fifth intercostal spaces).

- Dye volume: 20 mL distributed across injection sites.

- Outcomes: Dye distribution across intercostal spaces (T2-T6), accuracy of sonographic identification, and safety markers related to anatomical structures (e.g., internal thoracic artery).

Results

1. Dye distribution

   - Superficial PIP block: Triple injections (second, fourth, and fifth intercostal spaces) achieved consistent staining across all target spaces (T2-T6).

   - Deep PIP block: Double injections (third and fifth intercostal spaces) consistently covered T2-T6, outperforming single injections.

2. Sonographic findings

   - The transversus thoracis muscle, critical for deep PIP blocks, was reliably identified via ultrasound at the second to fifth intercostal spaces (agreement > 80%).

   - The internal thoracic artery was consistently located within 20 mm of the sternum, highlighting a safe zone for needle placement lateral to the artery.

3. Technique-specific observations

   - Superficial blocks require more injections to achieve widespread coverage due to the localized nature of dye spread.

   - Deep blocks offer broader craniocaudal distribution but carry a higher risk of pleural or vascular puncture without precise needle guidance.

Clinical implications

Optimizing PIP block techniques

- Superficial PIP block: Triple injections at the second, fourth, and fifth intercostal spaces are recommended to cover T2-T6.

- Deep PIP block: Double injections at the third and fifth intercostal spaces provide optimal dye spread with fewer needle passes.

Safety considerations

- Careful sonographic identification of the transversus thoracis muscle and internal thoracic artery is essential to avoid complications.

- To minimize vascular injury risks, ensure needle placement lateral to the midpoint between the sternum and costochondral junction.

Practical recommendations

- Tailor the injection technique based on procedural goals, prioritizing deep blocks for broader coverage and superficial blocks for targeted analgesia.

- Utilize real-time ultrasound to improve accuracy and safety in block performance.

Limitations and future directions

Study limitations

- Cadaveric findings may not fully translate to living patients due to differences in tissue dynamics and vascular flow.

- The study did not evaluate clinical outcomes, such as analgesic efficacy or patient-reported pain relief.

Future research

- Investigate the clinical effectiveness of the recommended techniques in surgical populations.

- Explore the impact of different local anesthetic volumes and concentrations on block success and duration.

Key takeaways

☑ Superficial PIP blocks require triple injections for consistent T2—T6 coverage, while deep PIP blocks achieve similar results with fewer injections.

☑ Ultrasound guidance is crucial for safe and effective PIP block administration, ensuring accurate identification of anatomical landmarks.

☑ These findings provide a foundation for refining clinical practices and optimizing analgesia in the chest wall and cardiac surgeries.

Additional recommended reading

1. Samerchua A, Leurcharusmee P, Supphapipat K, et al. Optimal techniques of ultrasound-guided superficial and deep parasternal intercostal plane blocks: A cadaveric study. *Reg Anesth Pain Med.* 2024;49:320-325.

2. Chin KJ, Versyck B, Pawa A. Ultrasound-guided fascial plane blocks of the chest wall: A state-of-the-art review. *Anaesthesia.* 2021;76(Suppl 1):110-126.

3. Schiavoni L, Cardetta F, Nenna A, et al. Parasternal intercostal nerve blocks in cardiac surgery: Evidence update and technical considerations. *J Cardiothorac Vasc Anesth.* 2022;36:4173-4182.

Combined rectus sheath and parasternal block in cardiac surgery

46

Why this topic is important

Postoperative pain following cardiac surgery, especially after midline sternotomy, is a significant challenge that can hinder recovery, impair respiratory function, and prolong hospital stays. Pain from sternotomy is compounded by the presence of chest drains in the epigastric region, which standard parasternal blocks (PSBs) may not adequately address. Uncontrolled pain often leads to shallow breathing, increasing the risk of pulmonary complications such as atelectasis and pneumonia. Effective pain management is, therefore, critical for promoting respiratory function, enabling early mobilization, and enhancing overall recovery.

While opioids are commonly used for postoperative analgesia, they come with considerable side effects like nausea, vomiting, and respiratory depression, which can delay recovery. Regional anesthesia techniques like PSB provide targeted pain relief and reduce opioid reliance, but they may not cover all sources of discomfort, particularly from chest drains. Combining a rectus sheath block (RSB) with PSB can potentially address this gap, offering comprehensive analgesia for both the sternotomy and epigastric regions. A recent study by Strulmia et al. investigates whether adding a rectus sheath block (RSB) to a parasternal block (PSB) can enhance pain control, reduce opioid use, and improve respiratory performance in cardiac surgery patients.

Objectives of this update

- To determine the analgesic benefits of combining RSB with PSB versus PSB alone with local infiltration at chest drain sites.

- To evaluate the impact of this combination on respiratory function and opioid consumption.

- To identify its potential to improve early postoperative recovery.

What is new

The randomized controlled trial by Strumia et al. 2024 demonstrates that adding RSB to PSB significantly reduces pain scores, improves respiratory performance, and decreases opioid-related side effects compared to PSB alone.

Key findings

Study design

- Participants: 58 patients undergoing cardiac surgery via midline sternotomy.

- Intervention groups:

  ○ Experimental group: Bilateral PSB + RSB.

  ○ Control group: Bilateral PSB + local infiltration of chest drain exit sites.

- Primary outcome: Pain at rest at extubation (Numeric Rate Scale [NRS]).

- Secondary outcomes: Pain during respiratory exercises, opioid consumption, respiratory performance, and side effects (e.g., postoperative nausea and vomiting [PONV]).

Results

1. Pain control:

   ○ Median NRS pain scores at extubation were significantly lower in the RSB group (4 vs. 5).

   ○ The pain remained lower at all subsequent time points in the RSB group, including during respiratory exercises.

2. Opioid consumption:

   ○ Median morphine use was reduced by 2 mg over 24 hours in the RSB group, with fewer patients requiring opioids (34.5% vs. 55%).

3. Respiratory performance:

   ○ At 6 and 12 hours post-extubation, the RSB group demonstrated improved inspiratory performance, lifting more spheres on the TriFlow incentive spirometer.

4. Side effects:

   ○ PONV occurred in only 7% of the RSB group compared to 34.5% in the control group.

Clinical implications

Benefits of combining RSB with PSB

- Enhanced analgesia: The combination relieves pain across the sternotomy and epigastric regions, improving patient comfort and recovery.

- Improved respiratory outcomes: Enhanced inspiratory function promotes better oxygenation and reduces the risk of pulmonary complications.

- Opioid-sparing strategy: Lower opioid consumption reduces side effects like PONV and may facilitate earlier mobilization.

Practical recommendations

- Use RSB alongside PSB for patients with epigastric drain placements to ensure comprehensive analgesia.

- Administer blocks with ultrasound guidance to maximize efficacy and minimize complications.

- Integrate multimodal analgesia to complement the benefits of regional blocks.

Limitations and future directions

Study limitations

- Lack of blinding for anesthesiologists performing blocks may introduce bias.

- The assessment was limited to 24 hours post-extubation, potentially missing longer-term effects.

Future research

- Explore the impact of this combination on hospital length of stay and long-term recovery.

- Investigate its efficacy in diverse cardiac surgical populations and outpatient settings.

Key takeaways

☑ Adding RSB to PSB reduces postoperative pain, improves respiratory performance, and minimizes opioid-related side effects in cardiac surgery patients.

☑ This combination is particularly effective for managing pain from epigastric drains.

☑ These findings support integrating RSB with PSB into routine analgesic protocols for cardiac surgeries involving midline sternotomy.

Additional recommended reading

1. Strumia A, Pascarella G, Sarubbi D, et al. Rectus sheath block added to parasternal block may improve postoperative pain control and respiratory performance after cardiac surgery: A superiority single-blinded randomized controlled clinical trial. *Reg Anesth Pain Med.* 2024;49:1-7.

2. Wang L, Jiang L, Jiang B, et al. Effects of Pecto-Intercostal Fascial block combined with rectus sheath block for postoperative pain management after cardiac surgery: A randomized controlled trial. *BMC Anesthesiol.* 2023;23:90.

3. Schiavoni L, Nenna A, Cardetta F, et al. Parasternal intercostal nerve blocks in patients undergoing cardiac surgery: Evidence update and technical considerations. *J Cardiothorac Vasc Anesth.* 2022;36:4173-82.

Accidental dural puncture and postdural puncture headache in obstetric anesthesia

47

Why this topic is important

Accidental dural puncture (ADP) and postdural puncture headache (PDPH) are recognized complications of neuraxial anesthesia in obstetric practice. Although often considered benign and self-limiting, ADP and PDPH can lead to serious chronic physical, neurological, and psychological sequelae, including postpartum depression, chronic headaches, and life-threatening complications like subdural hematomas. Raising awareness and enhancing the management of these conditions is critical to minimizing their long-term impact on maternal health.

Objectives of this update

- Discuss the incidence and risk factors for ADP and PDPH.

- Review the long-term physical, neurological, and psychological consequences of ADP and PDPH.

- Provide evidence-based guidance for the prevention, diagnosis, and management of these conditions.

What is new

- Evidence of chronic morbidity following PDPH, including persistent headaches, backache, and reduced breastfeeding rates.

- Increased recognition of life-threatening complications such as subdural hematoma (SDH) and cerebral venous thrombosis (CVT).

- Understanding of the psychological burden, including postpartum depression (PPD) and post-traumatic stress disorder (PTSD), associated with PDPH.

- Updated insights into risk factors, such as needle size, insertion technique, and maternal characteristics.

Incidence and risk factors

Incidence

- ADP occurs in 0.7-1.5% of obstetric epidural procedures.

- PDPH develops in 50-80% of cases following ADP, with the highest risk in young parturients.

Risk factors for ADP

- Needle Depth: Risk increases by 19% with each 1 cm increase in needle depth (specific to epidural procedures).

- Operator Experience: Higher rates in less experienced clinicians and during late shifts.

- Technique: Multiple attempts and needle rotation elevate the risk.

Risk factors for PDPH

- Maternal age: Younger age increases risk.

- Needle characteristics: Traumatic needles significantly elevate PDPH risk (specific to spinal anesthesia). Atraumatic 26G needles are preferable.

- Maternal BMI: Lower BMI may predispose to PDPH, though the evidence is mixed.

Pathophysiology and diagnosis

Pathophysiology

- CSF leakage: Results in intracranial hypotension and gravitational sagging of intracranial structures, leading to headache.

- Compensatory vasodilation: Reflex vasodilation due to intracranial pressure imbalance exacerbates headache.

Diagnosis

- PDPH typically presents within 24-72 hours of dural puncture, characterized by a dull, throbbing fronto-occipital headache exacerbated in the upright position and relieved by lying down.

- Associated symptoms: neck pain, photophobia, tinnitus, nausea, and dizziness.

Chronic and life-threatening consequences

Chronic morbidity

- Headache and backache: Persistent postural headaches (17.6-34.8%) and backaches (28-43.9%) are common.

- Psychological impact: High rates of postpartum depression (52%) and PTSD following PDPH. These are linked to decreased breastfeeding initiation and duration.

Neurological complications

- Subdural Hematoma (SDH): Caused by traction on intracranial veins. Symptoms include persistent headache, focal neurologic deficits, and vomiting.

- Cerebral Venous Thrombosis (CVT): Associated with decreased intracranial pressure and venous stasis, leading to seizures and motor weakness.

Rare complications

- Posterior reversible encephalopathy syndrome (PRES), bacterial meningitis, and pneumocephalus.

Prevention and management

Prevention

- Use atraumatic needles and minimize needle manipulation.

- Perform epidurals with experienced operators using proper techniques.

Accidental dural puncture and postdural puncture headache in obstetric anesthesia

Management

- Conservative: Bed rest, hydration, and analgesics.

- Epidural Blood Patch (EBP): Standard treatment for severe PDPH but must be used cautiously in cases of SDH or CVT to avoid worsening intracranial pressure (fig-1).

- Neurological monitoring: Persistent or worsening symptoms warrant imaging to rule out SDH or CVT.

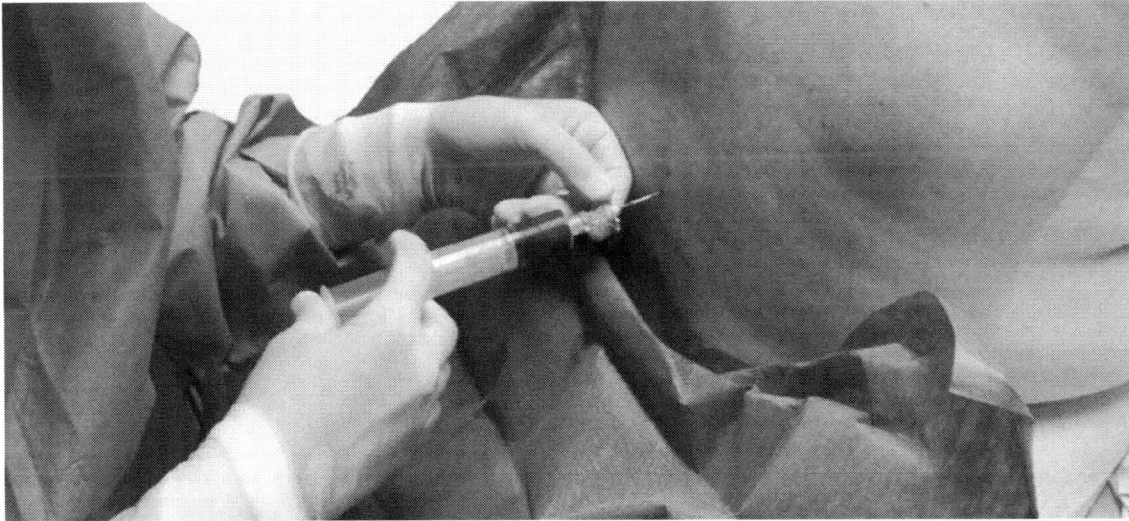

Fig-1. Administration of an epidural blood patch to treat postdural puncture headache. Blood is injected until a total volume of 20 mL is reached or the patient perceives significant pain or pressure in the back, whichever comes first.
Image taken from NYSORA LMS. https://nysoralms.com/

Key takeaways

- ☑ ADP and PDPH are often underestimated but can lead to significant chronic and life-threatening consequences.

- ☑ Persistent headaches, psychological disorders, and neurological complications demand vigilance and follow-up.

- ☑ Prevention strategies include using atraumatic needles and ensuring technical expertise during epidural placement.

- ☑ Multidisciplinary management, including early imaging and prompt treatment of complications, is crucial for optimizing outcomes.

Additional recommended reading

1. Armstrong S, Fernando R. Chronic consequences of accidental dural puncture and postdural puncture headache in obstetric anaesthesia. *Curr Opin Anesthesiol.* 2024;37(5):533-540.

2. Guglielminotti J, Landau R, Li G. Major neurologic complications associated with postdural puncture headache in obstetrics: a retrospective cohort study. *Anesth Analg.* 2019;129:1328-1336.

3. Orbach-Zinger S, Eidelman LA, Livne MY, et al. Long-term psychological and physical outcomes of women after postdural puncture headache: a retrospective cohort study. *Eur J Anaesthesiol.* 2021;38:130-137.

Regional anesthesia for pediatric and geriatric patients

Regional techniques in pediatric inguinal surgeries

48

Why this topic is important

Pediatric inguinal surgeries, such as inguinal hernia repair and orchidopexy, are among the most common procedures performed in children. Effective postoperative pain management in these surgeries is crucial to minimizing recovery complications, including delayed wound healing, prolonged hospitalization, and chronic pain. Inadequate pain control can negatively impact a child's immediate recovery and long-term pain perception.

Regional analgesia techniques, like caudal blocks, transversus abdominis plane (TAP) blocks, and quadratus lumborum (QL) blocks, have been widely used to provide opioid-sparing pain relief. Despite their popularity, the relative effectiveness of these techniques still needs to be determined. The systematic review and network meta-analysis by Hung et al. 2024 sought to evaluate the analgesic effects and safety profiles of regional blocks in pediatric inguinal surgeries.

Objectives of this update

- To determine the most effective regional analgesic technique for pain control in pediatric inguinal surgeries.

- To evaluate the duration of analgesia and opioid-sparing benefits of different regional blocks.

- To assess the safety and adverse event profiles of each technique.

What is new

The meta-analysis by Hung et al. 2024 included data from 69 randomized controlled trials (RCTs) involving 4636 pediatric patients. It provides a comparative analysis of the efficacy and safety of various regional blocks, offering clarity on the most effective strategies for managing postoperative pain in pediatric inguinal surgeries.

Study findings

Methodology

- Design: Systematic review and network meta-analysis of RCTs comparing regional analgesic techniques for pediatric inguinal surgeries.

- Participants: 4636 pediatric patients aged 0-18 years undergoing inguinal hernia repair, orchidopexy, or hydrocelectomy under general anesthesia.

- Techniques assessed:

  - Caudal block

  - TAP block

  - QL block

  - Ilioinguinal-iliohypogastric block (II-IHB; ultrasound-guided and landmark-based)

  - Wound infiltration (WI)

  - Systemic analgesia as a control

Key results

1. Time to first rescue analgesic

   - QL block had the longest duration of analgesia, delaying the need for rescue analgesics by an average of 7.7 hours compared to the control group.

   - TAP block also performed well, prolonging analgesia by 6.0 hours.

   - For orchidopexy, the caudal block was the only technique significantly extending analgesic duration (4.1 hours).

2. Rescue analgesic requirements

   - QL and TAP blocks significantly reduced the number of children needing rescue analgesics postoperatively compared to caudal block and WI.

3. Pain scores

   - QL and TAP blocks substantially reduced pain scores postoperatively during the first 12 hours.

4. Safety

   - No serious complications, such as neurological damage or systemic toxicity, were reported for any of the regional techniques.

   - Minor adverse effects included urinary retention (primarily with caudal blocks) and transient lower limb weakness.

Clinical implications

Optimizing pain control

The results strongly favor QL and TAP blocks for inguinal hernia repairs due to their extended analgesic duration and reduction in rescue analgesic needs. For orchidopexy, the caudal block remains the technique of choice, addressing specific pain patterns associated with the procedure.

Tailoring techniques to surgery type

- Inguinal hernia repair: QL and TAP blocks are optimal for their long-lasting analgesia and opioid-sparing effects.

- Orchidopexy: The caudal block is recommended due to its effectiveness in managing pain specific to scrotal incisions.

Safety considerations

While all techniques were safe, clinicians should monitor for urinary retention with caudal blocks and ensure proper needle placement for II-IHB and WI to minimize risks like vascular puncture.

Limitations

- Heterogeneity: Variations in surgical techniques, regional block protocols, and pain assessment methods introduce potential bias.

- Limited high-quality evidence: Many of the RCTs included in the analysis were assessed to have a high or moderate risk of bias, reducing confidence in some findings.

Key takeaways

☑ QL and TAP blocks provide the longest analgesia duration and superior pain control for inguinal hernia repairs.

☑ The caudal block is most effective for orchidopexy, extending analgesia for pain related to scrotal incisions.

☑ Regional techniques reduce opioid consumption, enhancing recovery and minimizing opioid-related risks.

☑ All techniques are safe, but caudal blocks may lead to urinary retention or transient motor weakness.

Additional recommended reading

1. Hung TY, Bai GH, Tsai MC, Lin YC. Analgesic effects of regional analgesic techniques in pediatric inguinal surgeries: A systematic review and network meta-analysis of randomized controlled trials. *Anesth Analg.* 2024;138(1):108-122.

2. Desai N, Chan E, El-Boghdadly K, Albrecht E. Caudal analgesia versus abdominal wall blocks for pediatric genitourinary surgery: systematic review and meta-analysis. *Reg Anesth Pain Med.* 2020;45:924-933.

3. Guay J, Suresh S, Kopp S. The use of ultrasound guidance for perioperative neuraxial and peripheral nerve blocks in children: a Cochrane review. *Anesth Analg.* 2017;124:948-958.

Dexamethasone as a perineural adjuvant for pediatric popliteal sciatic nerve block

49

Why this topic is important

Postoperative pain in pediatric foot and ankle surgeries can be moderate to severe, requiring effective management strategies to improve recovery and minimize opioid use. Popliteal sciatic nerve blocks are frequently employed for pain relief in these procedures, with ropivacaine being a common local anesthetic due to its prolonged duration and safety profile in children. However, the duration of these blocks often remains insufficient, leading to rebound pain. Dexamethasone, used as an adjuvant to local anesthetics, has shown promise in prolonging nerve block duration in adults. Yet, its efficacy and safety in young children, particularly concerning systemic effects such as blood glucose levels and inflammatory stress markers, remain unclear. A recent study by Reysner et al. 2024 investigates the potential benefits of perineural dexamethasone in pediatric nerve blocks, aiming to enhance postoperative pain management.

Objectives of this update

- To evaluate the effect of perineural dexamethasone on analgesia and motor block duration in pediatric sciatic nerve blocks.

- To assess secondary outcomes, including opioid consumption, stress markers (NLR and PLR), and blood glucose levels.

- To determine the safety of perineural dexamethasone in pediatric patients.

What is new

The study by Reynser et al. 2024 is one of the first randomized controlled trials (RCTs) to compare two doses of perineural dexamethasone (0.1 mg/kg and 0.05 mg/kg) in children, demonstrating significant prolongation of block duration and reduced opioid use without affecting glucose levels or stress markers.

Key findings

Study design and methodology

- Participants: 90 children aged 2-5 years undergoing foot or ankle surgery under spinal anesthesia.

- Intervention: Patients were randomized into three groups:

  ○ Control group: Ropivacaine 0.2% + saline.

  ○ DEX0.1 group: Ropivacaine 0.2% + dexamethasone 0.1 mg/kg.

  ○ DEX0.05 group: Ropivacaine 0.2% + dexamethasone 0.05 mg/kg.

- Outcomes: Time to first rescue opioid analgesia (primary outcome), motor block duration, pain scores, total opioid consumption, blood glucose, and stress markers (neutrophil-to-lymphocyte ratio [NLR] and platelet-to-lymphocyte ratio [PLR]).

Results

1. Time to first rescue opioid analgesia:

   - Significantly longer in the DEX0.1 group (18.4 ± 2.6 hours) compared to the DEX0.05 group (16.3 ± 2.8 hours) and the control group (8.5 ± 1.5 hours).

2. Motor block duration:

   - DEX0.1 significantly prolonged motor block duration (17.3 ± 2.5 hours) compared to DEX0.05 (15.2 ± 2.7 hours) and the control group (7.8 ± 1.1 hours).

3. Opioid consumption:

   - Total opioid use in the first 48 hours was lowest in the DEX0.1 group, with a significant reduction compared to the control group.

4. Pain scores (FLACC scale):

   - Lower pain scores were observed in the DEX0.1 group compared to the control group up to 20 hours post-surgery.

5. Blood glucose levels:

   - No significant differences were noted among groups at baseline, 24 hours, or 48 hours post-surgery.

6. Stress markers (NLR and PLR):

   - No significant differences were observed in NLR and PLR levels among the three groups.

7. Safety:

   - No nerve deficits or significant adverse events were reported in any group.

Clinical implications

Enhancing pediatric pain management

- Prolonged analgesia: Adding dexamethasone to ropivacaine significantly extends the duration of analgesia and reduces opioid consumption, offering better pain control in the critical postoperative period.

- Opioid-sparing benefits: Lower opioid use reduces the risk of associated side effects and dependency, which is particularly important in pediatric populations.

Safety profile of dexamethasone

- The study found no significant effects on blood glucose levels or surgical stress markers, indicating a favorable safety profile for dexamethasone at both doses tested.

Practical recommendations

- Preferred dose: A dose of 0.1 mg/kg is recommended for its superior efficacy in prolonging analgesia and motor block without additional risks.

- Monitoring: Standard postoperative monitoring suffices, as no systemic or local adverse effects were observed.

Limitations and future directions

Study limitations

- Blood glucose and stress markers were not assessed at intermediate time points (e.g., 6 or 12 hours), which could provide a more detailed understanding of dexamethasone's effects.

- The study was limited to children aged 2-5 years; results may not generalize to older pediatric populations or those with comorbidities.

Future research

- Explore the effects of dexamethasone with different local anesthetics or in older children.

- Investigate long-term outcomes, including chronic pain prevention and functional recovery.

Key takeaways

☑ Perineural dexamethasone significantly prolongs the duration of analgesia and motor block in pediatric sciatic nerve blocks.

☑ A 0.1 mg/kg dose provides optimal efficacy without impacting blood glucose levels or surgical stress markers.

☑ This adjuvant can enhance pain management in pediatric surgery while minimizing opioid requirements.

Additional recommended reading

1. Reysner M, Reysner T, Janusz P, et al. Dexamethasone as a perineural adjuvant to a ropivacaine popliteal sciatic nerve block for pediatric foot surgery: A randomized, double-blind, placebo-controlled trial. *Reg Anesth Pain Med.* 2024;49:1-7.

2. Veneziano G, Martin DP, Beltran R, et al. Dexamethasone as an adjuvant to femoral nerve block in children: A randomized controlled trial. *Reg Anesth Pain Med.* 2018;43:438-44.

3. Arafa SK, Elsayed AA, Hagras AM, et al. Pediatric postoperative pain control with quadratus lumborum block and dexamethasone: A clinical trial. *Pain Physician.* 2022;25:E987-98.

Value of nerve blocks by age and comorbidity

50

Why this topic is important

Peripheral nerve blocks (PNBs) are an integral component of pain management for total hip and knee arthroplasty (TJA), providing superior analgesia and reducing reliance on opioids. While the benefits of PNBs, such as improved pain control and reduced complication rates, are well-documented, questions remain about whether these effects vary across different patient demographics and health statuses.

As the aging population grows, the number of patients undergoing TJA with multiple comorbidities continues to rise. These patients have a higher baseline risk for perioperative complications, including respiratory compromise, acute renal failure, and delirium. Understanding how PNBs perform across subgroups defined by age and comorbidities is crucial for optimizing care strategies and targeting high-risk populations.

This update evaluates the findings of a nationwide study[1] across the USA assessing the differential impact of PNBs on perioperative outcomes in various age and comorbidity subgroups. It provides insights for clinicians tailoring anesthetic approaches in TJA patients.

Objectives of this update

- Examine the effects of PNBs on key outcomes like respiratory complications, renal failure, ICU admissions, and opioid use across age and comorbidity subgroups.

- Identify patient populations most likely to benefit from PNBs.

- Discuss the implications of these findings for clinical practice and anesthetic decision-making.

What is new

The study by Zhong et al. 2024 used a retrospective cohort analysis of 2.8 million TJA patients from the Premier Healthcare Database (2006-2019), stratifying outcomes by age and Charlson-Deyo comorbidity index categories (excellent, fair, poor).

Key findings

- PNBs were associated with reduced odds of postoperative respiratory complications, ICU admissions, prolonged hospital stays, and high opioid consumption, but the benefits varied by subgroup.

- Health status (comorbidity burden) was a stronger determinant of PNB efficacy than age.

- Compared to healthier subgroups, older adults with poor health ($\geq$ 3 comorbidities) experienced limited benefits from PNBs.

Detailed findings

Study design and methodology

- Population: 2,822,199 patients undergoing TJA (hip and knee) in U.S. hospitals.

- Intervention: PNB administration on the day of surgery, identified through billing codes.

- Subgroups: Patients were divided into six categories by age (< 65 vs. ≥ 65 years) and comorbidity burden (excellent: 0, fair: 1-2, poor: ≥ 3).

- Outcomes Assessed:

  - Respiratory complications

  - Acute renal failure

  - Delirium

  - ICU admissions

  - Prolonged length of stay (LOS)

  - High opioid consumption (> 426 mg oral morphine equivalents for knee TJA or > 372 mg for hip TJA)

Primary outcomes

1. Respiratory complications:

   - PNBs reduced respiratory complication odds in healthier subgroups.

   - No benefit was observed in the "poor" subgroups, highlighting a limited role for PNBs in mitigating respiratory risk in patients with significant comorbidities.

2. Acute renal failure:

   - Benefits were seen in all groups except Older Adults (Poor).

   - Reductions in renal failure may reflect improved pain control, reduced hemodynamic fluctuations, and lower opioid consumption.

3. ICU admissions:

   - PNBs significantly reduced ICU admissions in all groups except Older Adults (Poor),

suggesting composite benefits of reduced complications and improved recovery profiles.

4. Opioid consumption:

   - High opioid use was significantly lower in all subgroups except Adults (Poor).

   - This indicates that baseline opioid use patterns in sicker patients may limit the analgesic impact of PNBs.

5. Prolonged length of stay (LOS):

   - PNB use was associated with shorter LOS in Adults (Excellent), but no significant reductions were seen in other groups.

Implications for practice

Targeted use of PNBs

1. Maximizing benefits:

   - PNBs are most effective in younger and healthier patients or those with moderate comorbidities (Charlson-Deyo index 1-2).

   - For older, sicker patients, the benefits of PNBs may be marginal, and other strategies should be considered.

2. Risk-benefit considerations:

   - Avoid PNBs in patients with contraindications or poor health where efficacy may be limited.

   - Emphasize multimodal analgesia to complement PNBs, particularly in high-risk groups.

Integration into perioperative care

- Incorporate PNBs as part of enhanced recovery after surgery (ERAS) protocols, particularly for low- to moderate-risk patients.

- Use predictive tools to identify patients most likely to benefit from PNBs based on comorbidity burden and surgical risk factors.

Key takeaways

☑ PNBs reduce complications, resource utilization, and opioid use in TJA, with the greatest benefits in patients with low to moderate comorbidities.

☑ Health status is a stronger predictor of PNB efficacy than age, with limited benefits in older adults with significant comorbidities.

☑ Incorporating PNBs into ERAS protocols for targeted populations can optimize outcomes and resource use.

Additional recommended reading

1. Zhong H, Poeran J, Cozowicz C, et al. Does the impact of peripheral nerve blocks vary by age and comorbidity subgroups? A nationwide population-based study. *Reg Anesth Pain Med.* 2024;49:260-264.

2. Memtsoudis SG, Poeran J, Cozowicz C, et al. Peripheral nerve block anesthesia/analgesia for patients undergoing primary hip and knee arthroplasty. *Reg Anesth Pain Med.* 2021;46:971-85.

3. Deyo RA, Cherkin DC, Ciol MA. Adapting a clinical comorbidity index for use with administrative databases. *J Clin Epidemiol.* 1992;45:613-9.

Safety and risk management

Low-volume anesthetic with IV dexamethasone for superior trunk block and diaphragmatic paresis

51

Why this topic is important

Arthroscopic shoulder surgery often results in significant postoperative pain, requiring effective analgesic techniques for optimal recovery. While interscalene brachial plexus block is a common choice, its high incidence of diaphragmatic paresis (up to 100%) limits its use, especially in patients with compromised pulmonary function. The superior trunk block (STB) is a promising alternative, offering similar analgesic benefits with a lower risk of diaphragmatic paresis.

Reducing the volume of local anesthetic can further decrease the risk of phrenic nerve involvement, but this approach may shorten the analgesic duration. Adding intravenous dexamethasone, a known adjuvant for prolonging nerve block duration, offers a potential solution. A recent study by Kim et al.[1] evaluates whether combining low-volume local anesthetic with intravenous dexamethasone can provide effective analgesia while minimizing diaphragmatic paresis in patients undergoing arthroscopic shoulder surgery.

Objectives of this update

- To determine whether low-volume local anesthetic combined with intravenous dexamethasone reduces diaphragmatic paresis compared to conventional volume without dexamethasone.

- To assess the non-inferiority of analgesic duration with the low-volume approach.

- To evaluate secondary outcomes such as opioid consumption, pulmonary function, and patient satisfaction.

What is new

This randomized controlled trial by Kim et al. 2024 is the first to demonstrate that low-volume local anesthetic combined with intravenous dexamethasone significantly reduces diaphragmatic paresis while maintaining non-inferior analgesic duration compared to conventional volumes of local anesthetic without dexamethasone.

Study findings

Methodology

- Design: Randomized, controlled, non-inferiority trial with 84 adult patients undergoing arthroscopic shoulder surgery under general anesthesia.

- Groups:

  - Treatment group: 7 mL of 0.5% ropivacaine with 0.15 mg/kg intravenous dexamethasone.

  - Control group: 15 mL of 0.5% ropivacaine with intravenous saline.

- Primary outcomes:

  - Analgesic duration (time to first complaint of pain with Numeric Rating Scale ≥ 4).

  - The incidence of diaphragmatic paresis was assessed via M-mode ultrasonography.

- Secondary outcomes: Pain scores, total opioid consumption, pulmonary function, patient satisfaction, and postoperative nausea and vomiting (PONV).

Key results

1. Analgesic duration:

   - The time to first complaint of pain was similar between groups, demonstrating non-inferiority of the low-volume + dexamethasone approach compared to the conventional volume group.

   - The duration of the analgesic in the treatment group was 12.4 ± 6.8 hours versus 11.2 ± 4.6 hours in the control group.

   - The mean difference (-1.2 hours) was within the non-inferiority margin of 3 hours, confirming equivalent block efficacy.

2. Diaphragmatic paresis:

   - Diaphragmatic paresis occurred in 45.2% of the treatment group versus 85.4% in the control group, representing a 53% relative risk reduction.

   - This highlights the effectiveness of the low-volume approach in minimizing phrenic nerve involvement.

3. Secondary outcomes:

   - Opioid consumption: Total 24-hour opioid use was significantly lower in the treatment group (24.5 mg vs. 37.0 mg), reflecting an opioid-sparing benefit.

   - Pulmonary function: Despite reduced diaphragmatic paresis, pulmonary function (FEV1 and FEV6) did not significantly differ between groups.

   - Pain scores: Pain scores were similar overall, but the treatment group reported lower scores at 12 and 16 hours postoperatively, suggesting an intermediate-phase analgesic advantage.

   - PONV and patient satisfaction: PONV rates and patient satisfaction were comparable between groups. No block-related complications were reported in either group.

Comparison of low-volume anesthetic with IV dexamethasone vs. conventional volume for superior trunk block.

Variable	7 mL LA + IV Dexamethasone	15 mL LA (control group
Analgesic duration (hours)	12.4 ± 6.8	11.2 ± 4.6
Incidence of diaphragmatic paresis (%)	45.2	85.4
Opioid consumption (mg/ 24h)	45.2	37.0

Clinical implications

Advantages of low-volume STB with dexamethasone

- Reduced diaphragmatic paresis: Halving the incidence of diaphragmatic paresis makes this technique particularly beneficial for patients with pulmonary comorbidities.

- Non-inferior analgesic duration:
  Adding dexamethasone compensates for the shorter duration of analgesia typically associated with low-volume local anesthetics.

- Opioid-sparing effect:
  Reduced total opioid consumption enhances recovery and minimizes opioid-related side effects.

Practical considerations

- Technique feasibility: Ultrasound-guided STB is safe and reproducible, with minimal training requirements for experienced anesthesiologists.

- Patient selection: This option is ideal for patients at high risk of pulmonary complications or those undergoing ambulatory surgeries that require rapid recovery.

Key takeaways

- ☑ Combining low-volume local anesthetic with intravenous dexamethasone for STB reduces diaphragmatic paresis by over 50% compared to conventional volumes without dexamethasone.

- ☑ The technique provides non-inferior analgesic duration and reduces opioid consumption, supporting its role in multimodal analgesia.

- ☑ It particularly benefits patients at risk of pulmonary complications or requiring rapid recovery.

Additional recommended reading

1. Kim Y, Yoo S, Kim SH, et al. Comparison between low-volume local anesthetic with intravenous dexamethasone and conventional volume without dexamethasone for superior trunk block after arthroscopic shoulder surgery: A randomized controlled non-inferiority trial. *Reg Anesth Pain Med.* 2024;49:558-564.

2. Kim DH, Lin Y, Beathe JC, et al. Superior trunk block: A phrenic-sparing alternative to the interscalene block. *Anesthesiology.* 2019;131:521-33.

3. Baeriswyl M, Kirkham KR, Jacot-Guillarmod A, et al. Efficacy of perineural vs. systemic dexamethasone to prolong analgesia after peripheral nerve block: A meta-analysis. *Br J Anaesth.* 2017;119:183-91.

Perioperative management of anticoagulation: Best practices for Direct Oral Anticoagulants (DOACs)

52

Why this topic is important

Direct Oral Anticoagulants (DOACs) such as apixaban, rivaroxaban, edoxaban, and dabigatran, are indicated for conditions like stroke prevention in atrial fibrillation and the treatment or prevention of venous thromboembolism (VTE). DOACs are increasingly prescribed worldwide due to their advantages over traditional anticoagulants like warfarin, including fixed dosing, fewer drug interactions, and no need for routine coagulation monitoring.

As the population ages, the need for surgical or nonsurgical procedures in patients taking DOACs increases, with 20% of DOAC-treated individuals requiring some form of procedure each year. Managing anticoagulation in the perioperative setting is a complex but crucial task. Inappropriate management can lead to complications, either from excessive bleeding due to continued anticoagulation or from thromboembolic events if anticoagulation is interrupted incorrectly.

Ensuring that DOACs are handled appropriately in the perioperative period, particularly when balancing the risks of bleeding and thromboembolism, is critical to reducing perioperative morbidity and mortality. Anesthesiologists must carefully assess bleeding risks both before and after nerve blocks, as well as during catheter insertion or removal. Recent advances in clinical guidelines and standardized management protocols have provided clearer pathways to ensure safe outcomes for patients undergoing procedures while on DOAC therapy.

Objectives of this update

- To outline best practices for perioperative management of patients on DOACs.
- Describe risk-based approaches to stopping and restarting DOACs around surgical or nonsurgical procedures.
- To review emerging evidence and guidelines regarding DOAC reversal agents in urgent and emergent surgical settings.
- To highlight practical considerations for specific patient populations, such as those with kidney dysfunction or those requiring neuraxial anesthesia.

What is new

- Standardized protocols: New evidence-based protocols recommend stopping DOACs based on the procedure's bleeding risk, eliminating the need for routine coagulation tests in elective procedures.
- DOAC reversal agents: Idarucizumab (dabigatran-specific) and andexanet-α (Factor Xa inhibitors) are now recognized as effective in urgent or emergent surgical settings.
- Reduced heparin bridging: Unlike warfarin, DOACs do not require perioperative heparin bridging due to their shorter half-life and quicker resumption of anticoagulant effects postoperatively.
- Kidney dysfunction considerations: New guidelines emphasize adjusting the timing of DOAC discontinuation in patients with renal impairment to prevent excessive bleeding.

DOAC overview and pharmacology

DOACs inhibit either Factor Xa (apixaban, rivaroxaban, and edoxaban) or Factor IIa (dabigatran), leading to anticoagulant effects. The pharmacokinetics of DOACs include a rapid onset of action (2-3 hours post-ingestion) and relatively short half-lives (9-14 hours), with drug clearance primarily through the liver or kidneys.

Indications for low dose DOACs

- VTE prophylaxis after major orthopedic surgery (e.g., Hip or knee replacement).

- Extended prevention of recurrent deep vein thrombosis (DVT) and pulmonary embolism (PE).

- Acute coronary syndrome.

- Prevention of atherothrombotic events in symptomatic peripheral artery disease.

Indications for high dose DOACs

- Stroke prevention in nonvalvular atrial fibrilation.

- Acute venous thromboembolism treatment.

Clinical considerations

Due to these pharmacokinetic properties of DOACs, clinicians need to individualize perioperative anticoagulation management based on renal function, the timing of the procedure, and the overall bleeding risk.

DOAC	Typical low dose Dexamethasone	Typical high dose	Pharmacologic properties
Apixaban	2.5 mg BID	5 mg BID	A Factor Xa inhibitor with a half-life of 9-11 hours and 25% renal excretion.
Rivaroxaban	10 mg daily	20 mg daily	A Factor Xa inhibitor with a similar half-life (9-11 hours) but slightly higher renal clearance (33%).
Edoxaban	NA	60 mg daily	A Factor Xa inhibitor, with a half-life of 10-14 hours and about 50% renal excretion.
Dabigatran	220 mg daily	150 mg BID	A Factor IIa inhibitor with more reliance on kidney clearance (80%) and a longer half-life (12-14 hours and up to 24 hours in patients with renal impairment).

Perioperative DOAC management based on bleeding risk

The perioperative management of DOACs depends on the bleeding risk associated with the planned procedure. The key to effective management is understanding whether the procedure poses minimal, low-to-moderate, or high bleeding risk.

Minimal bleeding risk procedures

These include minor dental work, skin lesion removal, and cataract surgery. Patients undergoing such procedures generally do not need to interrupt their DOAC therapy. If there is a concern about bleeding, the morning dose of twice-daily DOACs (such as apixaban or dabigatran) can be omitted, or the once-daily DOACs (rivaroxaban or edoxaban) can be delayed until the evening following the procedure.

Low-to-moderate bleeding risk procedures

For procedures such as laparoscopic cholecystectomy, hernia repair, or gastrointestinal endoscopy with biopsy, the standard recommendation is to discontinue DOACs one day before surgery. This results in a 30-36 hour gap (about three half-lives of the drug) before the procedure, minimizing residual anticoagulation at the time of surgery. DOACs are then restarted the day after surgery, assuming hemostasis is secure.

High bleeding risk procedures

Major procedures, such as orthopedic joint replacements and major cancer surgeries pose a high risk of bleeding. For these patients, DOACs should be discontinued 2 days before surgery, creating a 60-68 hour interval (about five half-lives). DOACs can generally be resumed 48-72 hours postoperatively, depending on the patient's bleeding risk and surgical hemostasis.

Emergent and urgent procedures

Emergent procedures, such as those required for life-threatening conditions (e.g., ruptured abdominal aneurysm or major trauma), often need to be performed within 6 hours of presentation. There is no time to wait for the DOAC to wear off in these situations. In urgent surgeries (6-24 hours after presentation) or semi-urgent cases (24-48 hours), the decision-making process is similar but allows more time to measure DOAC levels if possible.

DOAC reversal in emergencies:

- Idarucizumab: A reversal agent specific to dabigatran, it neutralizes its anticoagulant effect rapidly and can be used when an immediate reversal is necessary.

- Andexanet-α: Reverses the anticoagulant effect of Factor Xa inhibitors (apixaban, rivaroxaban, and edoxaban). This agent is effective but expensive and has been associated with increased thrombotic risk.

- Prothrombin complex concentrates (PCC): These nonspecific reversal agents are also used in emergent situations for any DOAC. They are less expensive than specific reversal agents but may not be as effective.

In patients with high preoperative DOAC levels or when reversal agents are unavailable, delaying surgery may be recommended if feasible. In emergent cases, testing DOAC levels or using these reversal agents before surgery is advised.

Postoperative DOAC resumption

Timing of DOAC resumption postoperatively is just as important as preoperative discontinuation, as restarting anticoagulation too early increases the risk of surgical-site bleeding while delaying it too long increases the risk of thromboembolism.

For minimal or low-to-moderate risk procedures

DOACs can be resumed within 24 hours postoperatively if there are no signs of excessive bleeding. For minimal-risk procedures, like cataract surgery or minor dental work, resumption of DOACs can occur on the same day.

For high-risk procedures

In patients undergoing high bleeding risk surgeries (e.g., joint replacement, major cancer surgeries), DOAC resumption should be delayed until 48-72 hours postoperatively to reduce the risk of bleeding complications. Low-dose heparin (e.g., enoxaparin 40 mg daily) may be used during this waiting period to provide venous thromboembolism (VTE) prophylaxis until full-dose DOAC therapy can be safely resumed.

Special populations

Patients with impaired kidney function

Since the kidneys largely clear some DOACs (especially dabigatran), patients with renal impairment require special consideration. For patients with creatinine clearance (CrCl) less than 30 mL/min, dabigatran should be stopped earlier (3-4 days preoperatively). Apixaban, rivaroxaban, and edoxaban may also need longer cessation intervals depending on the severity of renal impairment.

Patients undergoing regional/ neuraxial anesthesia

Regional blocks are categorized into high-risk bleeding blocks (including neuraxial blocks, deep PNBs like infraclavicular, stellate ganglion, lumbar plexus, sciatic nerve blocks, etc.) and low-risk bleeding blocks (including superficial PNBs like interscalene, supraclavicular, axillary, transversus abdominus plane, femoral, ilio-inguinal, iliohypogastric Blocks, etc.).

Patients receiving spinal or epidural anesthesia are at higher risk of developing spinal hematomas if anticoagulation is not managed correctly. DOACs should generally be discontinued at least 72 hours before neuraxial procedures, and their resumption should be delayed until at least 48 hours after the procedure.

Table adapted from Kietaibl et al. (Joint ESAIC/ESRA guidelines, 2022).

DOAC	Last intake before neuraxial anesthesia in low-dose	Last intake before neuraxial anesthesia in high-dose
Rivaroxaban	24 hours	72 hours
Edoxaban	24 hours	72 hours
Apixaban	36 hours	72 hours
Dabigatran	48 hours	72 hours

Following neuraxial procedures, the next low dose of a DOAC should be administered in alignment with guidelines for postoperative VTE prophylaxis or therapeutic anticoagulation. For patients with neuraxial catheters, DOAC administration should be delayed until after catheter removal. In such cases, anticoagulation alternatives include low-dose LMWH or low-dose UFH.

Superficial nerve procedures may be performed at any DOAC dose, and the subsequent dose can be given at the regularly scheduled time. For deep nerve procedures, the same precautions and guidelines as those for neuraxial procedures should be followed.

In obstetric patients on DOAC therapy requiring neuraxial block, recommendations for the non-pregnant population apply.

If the minimum recommended therapy-free time interval has not elapsed, regional anesthesia decisions should consider the compressibility of the puncture site, proximity to large blood vessels, and involvement of neuraxial structures.

Key takeaways

☑ DOAC management should be tailored to the procedure's bleeding risk. Minimal-risk procedures generally do not require interruption, while higher-risk procedures require discontinuation of DOACs 1-2 days before the surgery.

☑ DOACs can typically be restarted 24-72 hours postoperatively, depending on the risk of postoperative bleeding.

☑ Reversal agents like idarucizumab and andexanet-α are essential for managing patients requiring emergent surgery, though their high cost and potential thrombotic risks need careful consideration.

☑ Routine testing of DOAC levels is not necessary for elective procedures but may be useful in urgent or emergent cases.

☑ Renal function and anesthesia type are important factors to consider in the perioperative management of DOACs, with adjustments to timing needed in special populations.

Additional recommended reading

1. Douketis JD, Spyropoulos AC. Perioperative management of patients taking direct oral anticoagulants: *A Review. JAMA.* 2024;332(10):825-834.

2. Douketis JD, Spyropoulos AC, Murad MH, et al. Perioperative management of antithrombotic therapy: An American College of Chest Physicians clinical practice guideline. *Chest.* 2022;162(5).

3. Kietaibl S, Ferrandis R, Godier A, et al. Regional anesthesia in patients on antithrombotic drugs: joint ESAIC/ESRA guidelines. *Eur J Anaesthesiol.* 2022;39(2):100-132.

4. Horlocker TT, Vandermeulen E, Kopp SL, Gogarten W, Leffert LR, Benzon HT. Regional Anesthesia in the Patient Receiving Antithrombotic or Thrombolytic Therapy: American Society of Regional Anesthesia and Pain Medicine Evidence-Based Guidelines (Fourth Edition). *Reg Anesth Pain Med.* 2018 Apr;43(3):263-309.

Special considerations in neuraxial anesthesia

Spinal hematoma case reports

53

Why this topic is important

Spinal epidural hematomas (SEH) are rare but potentially catastrophic complications associated with trauma, coagulopathy, and neuraxial interventions. These hematomas can cause significant neurological deficits, including paralysis, if not identified and managed promptly. With the increasing use of neuraxial and interventional pain procedures, particularly in patients on anticoagulants, understanding the risk factors, presentation, and outcomes of SEH is critical.

The American Society of Regional Anesthesia and Pain Medicine (ASRA) guidelines aim to mitigate these risks in patients receiving anticoagulation. However, SEH can occur even when guidelines are followed. A recent comprehensive review by Benzon et al. 2024 examines case reports across diverse populations-including pediatric, obstetric, and adult patients-to identify trends in causation, adherence to guidelines, and predictors of recovery.

Objectives of this update

- Summarize the causes and risk factors for spinal epidural hematomas in different patient populations.

- Evaluate neurological outcomes in relation to the degree of neurological deficit and timing of surgical intervention.

- Highlight the implications of guideline adherence and the need for vigilant monitoring.

What is new

This study reviewed 940 cases of SEH across pediatric, obstetric, and adult populations. It is the first to analyze such a large dataset and assess outcomes based on neurological status, surgical timing, and adherence to anticoagulation guidelines.

Key findings:

- Spontaneous SEH accounted for a significant proportion of cases, especially in pediatric and non-obstetric adult populations.

- SEH occurred even with ASRA guideline adherence, particularly in patients on multiple anticoagulants.

- Neurological recovery was more strongly associated with preoperative neurological status than with the timing of surgical decompression.

Detailed findings

Study design

PubMed and Embase databases to examine 940 case reports published between 1954 and 2022. The cases were stratified into pediatric, obstetric (OB), and adult (non-OB) populations, with further subdivision by anticoagulant use. Recovery was assessed based on the American Spinal Injury Association (ASIA) Impairment Scale and timing of surgery.

Primary outcomes: Causation and recovery

1. Causative factors:

   - Pediatric: Most cases were spontaneous, linked to trauma or coagulation disorders (e.g., hemophilia).

   - Obstetric: SEH occurred postpartum or during the third trimester, often related to neuraxial procedures.

   - Adult non-OB:
     Spontaneous cases predominated, with trauma, neuraxial procedures, and interventional pain treatments contributing to others.

2. Adherence to guidelines:

   - SEH occurred despite adherence to ASRA guidelines, particularly in patients on multiple anticoagulants.

   - Deviations from guidelines included inadequate discontinuation of anticoagulants or inappropriate timing of neuraxial procedures.

3. Neurological recovery:

   - Recovery was closely associated with preoperative ASIA grade, with ASIA D patients demonstrating the highest likelihood of full recovery.

   - Timing of surgery (< 12 hours vs. > 48 hours) had minimal impact on outcomes, challenging the traditional emphasis on early intervention.

Secondary findings

Pediatric and obstetric populations

- Pediatric patients:

  - Hemophilia and sports-related trauma were common causes.

  - 60% achieved full recovery, often with prompt surgical decompression.

- Obstetric cases:

  - SEH was often linked to epidural placement or removal, with 57% achieving full recovery.

  - Coagulopathy during pregnancy contributed to several cases.

Adult non-obstetric populations

- Patients on anticoagulants:

  - SEH was often spontaneous, especially in those on multiple agents (e.g., warfarin and low molecular weight heparin).

  - Adherence to ASRA guidelines reduced risk but did not eliminate SEH occurrence.

- Patients not on anticoagulants:

  - Trauma and spontaneous cases dominated.

  - Recovery outcomes were similar to those in anticoagulated patients when matched by ASIA grade.

Management strategies

- Surgical decompression:

  - Most effective in ASIA C and D patients.

  - The timing of surgery (< 12 hours vs. > 48 hours) was less critical than preoperative neurological status.

- Conservative management:

  - Effective for ASIA C-E patients, with spontaneous recovery noted in some ASIA A patients.

Implications for practice

Patient safety and guideline adherence

1. Anticoagulation management:

   ◦ ASRA guidelines should be strictly followed, with heightened caution for patients on multiple anticoagulants.

   ◦ Vigilant monitoring during and after neuraxial procedures is crucial, even with guideline adherence.

2. Neurological assessment:

   ◦ Preoperative ASIA grading should guide the urgency of surgical intervention.

   ◦ Frequent neurological checks may help identify candidates for conservative management.

Surgical timing

- The lack of a clear relationship between surgical timing and recovery challenges the traditional emphasis on immediate intervention.

- Optimizing patient condition and maintaining close monitoring may be preferable to rushed decompression.

Key takeaways

☑ Spinal epidural hematomas are rare but can occur spontaneously or in association with trauma, coagulopathy, and neuraxial procedures.

☑ Adherence to ASRA guidelines reduces SEH risk but does not eliminate it, particularly in patients on multiple anticoagulants.

☑ Preoperative neurological status is the strongest predictor of recovery, surpassing the impact of surgical timing.

☑ Vigilant monitoring and individualized risk assessment are essential for optimizing outcomes.

Additional recommended reading

1. Benzon HT, Nelson AM, Patel AG, et al. Literature review of spinal hematoma case reports: causes and outcomes in pediatric, obstetric, neuraxial and pain medicine cases. *Reg Anesth Pain Med.* 2024;49:1-7.

2. Horlocker TT, Vandermeulen E, Kopp SL, et al. Regional anesthesia in the patient receiving antithrombotic or thrombolytic therapy: ASRA evidence-based guidelines. *Reg Anesth Pain Med.* 2018;43:263-309.

3. Kreppel D, Antoniadis G, Seeling W. Spinal hematoma: a literature survey with meta-analysis of 613 patients. *Neurosurg Rev.* 2003;26:1-49.

Neuraxial anesthesia and arachnoiditis: A review of evidence and risks

54

Why this topic is important

Arachnoiditis is a rare but debilitating condition characterized by inflammation and scarring of the pia-arachnoid. It can lead to neurological deficits ranging from pain and weakness to paraplegia. Neuraxial anesthesia (fig-1), commonly used for pain management and surgical procedures, has been implicated as a potential cause of arachnoiditis due to local anesthetic neurotoxicity. A recent review by Brenn et al. 2024 examines the evidence linking neuraxial local anesthetics to arachnoiditis, aiming to clarify risks and guide prevention strategies. While arachnoiditis is infrequent, its severe consequences necessitate a thorough understanding of the potential role of local anesthetics and other contributory factors such as procedural complications, preservatives, and additives.

Objectives of this update

- To summarize evidence regarding the association between neuraxial local anesthetics and arachnoiditis.

- To identify procedural and pharmacological risk factors contributing to neurotoxicity.

- To highlight gaps in knowledge and implications for clinical practice.

What is new

This review by Brenn et al. 2024 analyzed 38 studies spanning 80 years. It emphasizes the inconsistent and incomplete nature of reported cases and highlights confounding factors that obscure the true relationship between local anesthetics and arachnoiditis.

Study findings

Methodology

- Study design: Systematic narrative review of published case reports and case series from 1942 to 2022.

- Data sources: MEDLINE, Embase, CINAHL, and Cochrane CENTRAL.

- Inclusion criteria: Reports describing cases of arachnoiditis following neuraxial anesthesia attributed to local anesthetic neurotoxicity.

38 articles were included, encompassing 130 cases. Most studies involved single-case reports or small case series, often lacking critical procedural details.

Key results

1. Procedural characteristics

   ◦ Neuraxial techniques included epidurals (60%), spinals (37%), and combined spinal-epidurals (3%).

   ◦ Obstetrical cases accounted for 44% of procedures.

   ◦ At least 57% of cases reported procedural complications such as multiple attempts or pain during needle insertion.

2. Local anesthetic agents

   ◦ Only 51% of reports specified the type of local anesthetic used, with bupivacaine, lidocaine, and chloroprocaine being the most common.

   ◦ In some cases, excessive dosing and preservative-containing solutions were noted, though often without sufficient detail to establish causation.

3. Neurological outcomes

   ◦ Symptoms of arachnoiditis ranged from back and leg pain to severe motor and sensory deficits.

   ◦ Symptom onset varied widely, from immediate to as long as eight years post-procedure.

   ◦ Outcomes were heterogeneous: partial recovery was most common, while complete recovery was rare.

4. Reporting inconsistencies

   ◦ Only 56% of essential procedural details were consistently reported.

   ◦ Details on preservatives, additives, and needle specifications should have been more frequently included.

Clinical implications

Risk factors and prevention

- Procedural complications: Pain, paresthesia, or multiple needle passes during neuraxial anesthesia may increase the risk of arachnoiditis. Improved technique and ultrasound guidance could reduce these complications.

- Preservative use: Neuraxial injections should preferentially use preservative-free formulations to minimize chemical irritation.

- Dosing considerations: Avoidance of excessive dosing and adherence to guidelines for local anesthetic concentration and volume are crucial.

Enhancing informed consent

Given the potential for arachnoiditis and its devastating consequences, patients should be informed about this rare complication during consent discussions for neuraxial anesthesia.

Limitations

- Data quality: Many reports were outdated and lacked essential procedural details, limiting their relevance to modern practice.

- Confounding factors: The role of antiseptics, additives, and preexisting conditions often needed to be clarified.

Key takeaways

☑ The association between neuraxial local anesthetics and arachnoiditis needs to be better characterized, with outdated and incomplete data dominating the literature.

☑ Procedural complications, preservative use, and excessive dosing may contribute to neurotoxicity, but clear causative links remain elusive.

☑ Improved procedural techniques, preservative-free formulations, and strict adherence to dosing guidelines are essential to mitigate risks.

☑ Future research should focus on high-quality, prospective data collection and reporting to clarify the pathophysiology and prevention of arachnoiditis.

Additional recommended reading

1. Brenna CTA, Khan S, Poots C, et al. Association between perioperative neuraxial local anesthetic neurotoxicity and arachnoiditis: A narrative review of published reports. *Reg Anesth Pain Med.* 2024;49:726-750.

2. Rice MJ, Hu P, Rosenquist RW. Lack of association between obstetrical epidurals and arachnoiditis: A systematic review. *Reg Anesth Pain Med.* 2005;30(3):237-242.

3. Hooten WM, Eldrige JS, Smith WR. Arachnoiditis: Mechanisms, diagnosis, and management. *Reg Anesth Pain Med.* 2015;40(4):439-445.

Failed spinal anesthesia for cesarean delivery

55

Why this topic is important

Spinal anesthesia (SA) is the preferred technique for cesarean delivery (CD) due to its reliability, rapid onset, and minimal impact on neonatal outcomes. However, failure of spinal anesthesia-defined as inadequate analgesia necessitating supplementation or conversion to general anesthesia (GA) poses significant challenges.

Failed spinal anesthesia can lead to intraoperative pain, patient dissatisfaction, medicolegal issues, and delayed surgical care. The incidence of SA failure ranges from 2% to 12%, depending on the definition and patient population. Identifying and managing these failures are crucial to ensuring maternal comfort and safety. Moreover, the emotional significance of CD as a major life event underscores the need for optimal anesthetic care.

This update synthesizes recent insights into the prevention, identification, and management of failed spinal anesthesia for CD, focusing on technical, pharmacological, and patient-centered strategies.

Objectives of this update

- Understand the incidence and risk factors for failed spinal anesthesia during CD.

- Evaluate methods for identifying inadequate neuraxial blocks preoperatively and intraoperatively.

- Discuss evidence-based management strategies, including repeat neuraxial and general anesthesia options.

What is new

Recent findings include:

- Identification of key risk factors such as prior cesarean delivery, low gestational age, and prolonged surgical duration.

- Clarification of the mechanisms underlying failed SA, including pseudo-successful lumbar punctures and inadequate intrathecal dosing.

- Development of structured algorithms for block testing, repeat spinal procedures, and intraoperative pain management.

Incidence of failed spinal anesthesia

- Retrospective studies report failure rates ranging from 2.1% to 10.2%, with variability influenced by definitions of failure (e.g., need for GA, supplementary analgesia).

- Real-world failure rates exceed guideline benchmarks, such as the Royal College of Anaesthetists' recommendation of < 1% conversion to GA for elective CD.

Risk factors for failed spinal anesthesia

1. Patient-specific factors:

   ◦ Prior cesarean delivery

   ◦ Low gestational age and birth weight: Associated with insufficient intrathecal drug spread due to anatomical and physiological differences.

   ◦ Body Mass Index (BMI): Lower BMI is a risk factor.

2. Technical factors:

   ◦ The use of smaller-gauge needles (e.g., 27G vs. 25G) increases failure risk.

   ◦ Punctures at lower lumbar levels (L4/5) are associated with higher failure rates, likely due to limited drug spread.

3. Procedure-related factors:

   ◦ Longer surgical duration and the addition of procedures (e.g., tubal ligation) increase the likelihood of failure.

   ◦ Emergency CD settings may compromise block efficacy due to time constraints and suboptimal technique.

Prevention strategies

1. Optimizing technique:

   ◦ Meticulous patient positioning and precise identification of the subarachnoid space.

   ◦ Verification of drug preparation and dosing, especially for preterm or low birth weight pregnancies.

   ◦ Use of combined spinal-epidural (CSE) anesthesia for anticipated longer surgeries.

2. Block testing:

   ◦ Motor block evaluation (e.g., straight leg raise test) should precede sensory level testing.

   ◦ A T5 level to loss of touch sensation is mandatory before surgical incision.

3. Prophylactic interventions:

   ◦ Intrathecal adjuvants like fentanyl or sufentanil enhance block quality.

   ◦ Avoid over-reduction in intrathecal dosing for preterm or low-weight pregnancies to prevent inadequate spread.

Management of failed spinal anesthesia

1. Preoperative failure:

   ◦ Repeat spinal anesthesia: Safe in cases of complete block failure but requires reduced dosing to minimize risks of high spinal block.

   ◦ Conversion to epidural: Consider transitioning to epidural anesthesia for partial failures, particularly in labor epidural augmentation scenarios.

2. Intraoperative failure:

   ◦ Early pain (pre-delivery): Transition to GA when intravenous opioids are insufficient.

- Late pain (post-delivery): Options include wound infiltration with local anesthetics or intra-abdominal chloroprocaine instillation.

- Reassure and involve patients in decision-making to mitigate psychological distress.

3. Systemic analgesic support:

- IV boluses of fast-acting opioids (e.g., remifentanil 20 µg) are first-line interventions for intraoperative pain.

- Adjuncts like ketamine or nitrous oxide may be considered in appropriate clinical contexts.

- Use clear communication to align patient expectations with clinical realities.

2. Postoperative follow-up:

- Address intraoperative pain experiences during follow-up to identify areas for improvement and provide psychological support.

System-level improvements

1. Training and guidelines:

- Enhance provider education on testing blocks and recognizing failure.

- Implement written protocols for failed spinal anesthesia management.

2. Documentation:

- Record all block assessments, patient-reported pain, and management interventions to ensure continuity of care and medico-legal compliance.

Implications for practice

Patient-centered care

1. Informed consent:

- Discussions should include the possibility of block failure and alternative strategies, including GA.

Key takeaways

☑ Failed spinal anesthesia for cesarean delivery occurs in up to 12% of cases and requires tailored prevention and management strategies.

☑ Risk factors include prior cesarean delivery, lower BMI, and technical challenges during block placement.

☑ Management includes repeating neuraxial procedures with caution, systemic analgesia, or conversion to GA, depending on surgical progress.

☑ Patient-centered communication and meticulous documentation are essential for quality care and safety.

Additional recommended reading

1. Girard T, Savoldelli GL. Failed spinal anesthesia for cesarean delivery: prevention, identification and management. *Curr Opin Anesthesiol.* 2024;37:207-212.

2. Patel R, Kua J, Sharawi N, et al. Inadequate neuraxial anesthesia in patients undergoing elective cesarean section: A systematic review. *Anaesthesia.* 2022;77:598-604.

3. Stav M, Matatov Y, Hoffmann D, et al. Incidence of conversion to general anesthesia and need for intravenous supplementation in parturients undergoing cesarean section under spinal anesthesia: A retrospective observational study. *Acta Anaesthesiol Scand.* 2023;67:29-35.

Impact of spinal and epidural anesthesia on perioperative outcomes in noncardiac surgery

56

Why this topic is important

Spinal and epidural anesthesia (neuraxial techniques) are pivotal in modern anesthesia and acute pain management. While their immediate effects on nociceptive and sympathetic pathways are evident in clinical practice, their broader impact on perioperative outcomes remains a subject of ongoing investigation. With the rise of minimally invasive surgeries and enhanced recovery protocols, the relevance of neuraxial techniques in optimizing patient-centered outcomes is increasingly debated. A recent review by Hewson et al. 2024 synthesizes recent evidence on the impact of spinal and epidural anesthesia on perioperative outcomes, such as pulmonary complications, mortality, and patient comfort in adult noncardiac surgery.

Objectives of this update

- To evaluate the effect of neuraxial anesthesia on key patient-centered perioperative outcomes.

- To compare evidence supporting neuraxial anesthesia versus general anesthesia for noncardiac surgery.

- To provide insights for clinical decision-making in anesthetic planning.

What is new

This review by Hewson et al. 2024, encompassing data from 2018 to 2023, highlights recent findings that underscore the benefits of neuraxial anesthesia in patient comfort and mortality reduction, especially in major open thoracoabdominal surgeries. However, evidence supporting its role in other domains, such as cancer outcomes and renal function, is less consistent.

Key findings

Patient comfort and postoperative outcomes

- Neuraxial anesthesia consistently improves pain control, reducing postoperative opioid consumption and incidence of nausea and vomiting (PONV).

- For lower limb arthroplasty, spinal anesthesia showed reduced hospital length of stay and opioid use but increased risks of pruritus and transient neurologic symptoms when intrathecal opioids were used.

Pulmonary complications

- Epidural analgesia reduced risks of pneumonia, atelectasis, and respiratory failure in major thoracoabdominal surgeries.

- Meta-analyses reveal reduced postoperative pulmonary complication rates with thoracic epidurals, with benefits attenuating in recent years due to advances in surgical and anesthetic care.

Mortality outcomes

- Epidural analgesia was associated with lower 30-day and 90-day mortality after emergency abdominal surgeries, likely through enhanced recovery and reduced pulmonary complications.

- In elective surgeries, meta-analyses show a survival benefit with neuraxial anesthesia in frail populations undergoing major orthopedic procedures.

Inconsistent evidence in other domains

1. Infection and sepsis

   - Observational data suggest neuraxial techniques may lower surgical site infections (SSIs) through improved immune function and reduced stress responses.

   - However, randomized trials have not confirmed this finding.

2. Postoperative cancer outcomes

   - Mechanistic studies suggest potential benefits of neuraxial anesthesia in preserving immune function and reducing tumor recurrence.

   - Recent trials fail to demonstrate survival benefits or reduced cancer progression rates.

3. Renal outcomes

   - While retrospective studies indicate a reduced incidence of acute kidney injury (AKI) with neuraxial techniques, robust prospective data are lacking.

4. Cardiovascular outcomes

   - Evidence of reduced perioperative myocardial infarction rates with thoracic epidurals exists in high-risk populations, but findings are inconsistent across other surgical cohorts.

Clinical implications

Benefits in specific surgeries

- Thoracoabdominal surgery:
  Epidurals provide superior pain control and reduce complications, maintaining their role as a standard analgesic technique.

- Laparoscopic procedures: Alternatives such as transversus abdominis plane (TAP) and quadratus lumborum blocks may suffice due to lower risk profiles.

- Orthopedic procedures:
  Neuraxial anesthesia offers notable benefits in frail patients, supporting its use in hip and knee arthroplasty.

Balancing risks and benefits

- Risks such as hypotension, urinary retention, and rare neurological complications must be considered.

- Tailored approaches integrating patient comorbidities and surgical risks are essential for optimizing outcomes.

Limitations

Study limitations

- High variability in study designs and outcome measures limits direct comparisons.

- Observational studies dominate the literature, with fewer randomized trials to confirm causation.

Key takeaways

☑ Neuraxial anesthesia improves postoperative comfort, reduces opioid consumption, and lowers pulmonary complication risks, particularly in major open surgeries.

☑ Survival benefits are evident in specific high-risk populations but not universal across all procedures.

☑ Evidence supporting its impact on cancer, renal, and infection outcomes remains inconclusive.

☑ Clinical decision-making should balance benefits against risks and be guided by patient and surgical factors.

Additional recommended reading

1. Hewson DW, Tedore TR, Hardman JG. Impact of spinal or epidural anaesthesia on perioperative outcomes in adult noncardiac surgery: a narrative review of recent evidence. *Br J Anaesth.* 2024;133(2):380-399.

2. Neuman MD, Elkassabany NM, Eckenhoff RG. Regional versus general anesthesia in elderly patients undergoing major surgery. *J Am Geriatr Soc.* 2020;68(3):591-595.

3. Popping DM, Elia N, Marret E, et al. Protective effects of epidural analgesia on pulmonary complications after abdominal and thoracic surgery: a meta-analysis. *Arch Surg.* 2008;143(10):990-999.

Efficacy of ultrasound guidance versus anatomical landmarks for neuraxial puncture

57

Why this topic is important

Neuraxial anesthesia techniques, including spinal, epidural, and combined spinal-epidural anesthesia, are essential for various surgical and diagnostic procedures. Traditionally performed using anatomical landmarks, neuraxial punctures often have variable success rates, particularly in obese patients (fig-1) or those with challenging anatomy. The first-pass success rate with traditional methods is only 60-70%, which can impact patient satisfaction, procedural efficiency, and complication rates.

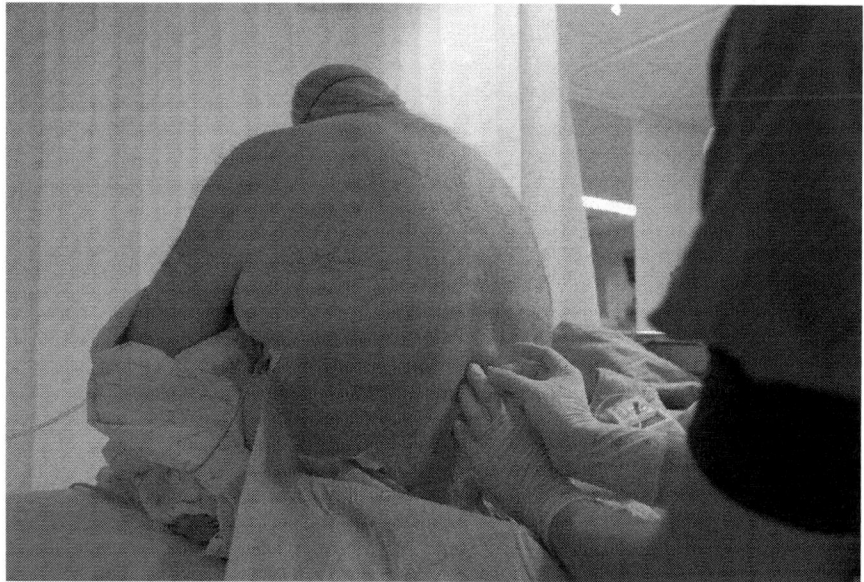

Fig-1. Spinal anesthesia in an obese patient.
Image taken from NYSORA LMS. https://nysoralms.com/

Ultrasound guidance has emerged as a promising alternative to anatomical landmark techniques, potentially improving success rates, reducing complications, and enhancing patient comfort. However, the optimal ultrasound-guided method-whether preprocedural, real-time, or computer-aided-remains unclear.

This update evaluates evidence comparing ultrasound guidance with anatomical landmarks for neuraxial punctures, focusing on first-pass success, patient satisfaction, and procedure times.

Objectives of this update

- Compare the efficacy of ultrasound guidance and anatomical landmark techniques for neuraxial punctures.

- Analyze the benefits of different ultrasound-guided methods: preprocedural, real-time, and computer-aided approaches.

- Provide guidance for clinical application and future research priorities.

What is new

A systematic review and network meta-analysis of 74 randomized controlled trials involving 7,090 patients assessed:

- First-pass success rates: Ultrasound guidance outperformed anatomical landmarks, with preprocedural and real-time techniques showing the highest success rates.

- Patient satisfaction: Preprocedural ultrasound increased satisfaction scores compared to landmark techniques, although evidence was of low confidence.

- Safety: Ultrasound guidance was associated with fewer complications, such as unintentional dural punctures and paraesthesia.

Detailed findings

Methods

The meta-analysis evaluated four techniques:

1. Preprocedural ultrasound: Used to mark needle insertion points and measure skin-to-epidural space distance.

2. Real-time ultrasound: Enables continuous visualization of the needle during insertion.

3. Computer-aided ultrasound: Provides automated three-dimensional imaging to identify neuraxial landmarks.

4. Anatomical landmarks: Traditional palpation-based approach.

Primary outcomes

1. First-pass success:

   ○ Real-time ultrasound: Highest success rate (risk ratio [RR] 1.9).

   ○ Preprocedural ultrasound: Also significantly improved success compared to landmarks (RR 1.6).

   ○ Computer-aided ultrasound: Increased success, though evidence was less precise (RR 1.8).

2. Patient satisfaction:

   ○ Preprocedural ultrasound yielded slightly higher satisfaction scores compared to landmarks (standardized mean difference 0.28.

   ○ Real-time and computer-aided methods showed minimal differences in satisfaction.

3. Procedure time:

   ○ Ultrasound-guided techniques had comparable procedure times to landmarks, indicating feasibility without prolonging workflow.

Safety outcomes

- Ultrasound-guided methods reduced adverse events, such as:

   ○ Unintentional dural punctures: 0-5% with preprocedural ultrasound versus up to 6.7% with landmarks.

   ○ Paraesthesia: Lower incidence with ultrasound methods compared to landmarks.

Implications for practice

Advantages of ultrasound guidance

1. Improved success rates:

   ○ Ultrasound increases accuracy, especially in challenging cases like obesity or anatomical abnormalities.

2. Enhanced safety:

   ○ Fewer needle redirections and reduced risk of complications.

3. Patient comfort:

   ○ Better first-pass success translates to less procedural discomfort and higher satisfaction.

Technique selection

- Preprocedural ultrasound: Recommended for routine use due to ease of implementation, minimal training requirements, and high success rates.

- Real-time ultrasound:
  Useful for complex cases requiring precise visualization but requires advanced skills and equipment.

- Computer-aided ultrasound:
  Emerging technology with potential for rapid adoption but limited evidence to date.

Training considerations

- Training operators to perform ultrasound-guided neuraxial procedures improves outcomes after 22-36 scans, highlighting the importance of structured education.

Challenges and limitations

1. Heterogeneity of studies:

   ° Variation in patient populations, procedures, and outcome definitions complicates data interpretation.

2. Operator expertise:

   ° Success rates vary significantly depending on operator's experience with ultrasound.

3. Resource limitations:

   ° High-quality ultrasound equipment may not be available in all settings.

Key takeaways

☑ Ultrasound guidance, especially preprocedural and real-time methods, improves first-pass success rates for neuraxial punctures compared to anatomical landmarks.

☑ Ultrasound-guided techniques are safe, feasible, and associated with higher patient satisfaction.

☑ Preprocedural ultrasound offers the best balance of simplicity, effectiveness, and accessibility.

☑ Operator training is essential to maximize the benefits of ultrasound-guided neuraxial techniques.

Additional recommended reading

1. Kamimura Y, Yamamoto N, Shiroshita A, et al. Comparative efficacy of ultrasound guidance versus conventional anatomical landmarks for neuraxial puncture in adult patients: A systematic review and network meta-analysis. *Br J Anaesth.* 2024;132(5):1097-1111.

2. Shaikh F, Brzezinski J, Alexander S, et al. Ultrasound imaging for lumbar punctures and epidural catheterizations: Systematic review and meta-analysis. *BMJ.* 2013;346:f1720.

3. Perlas A, Chaparro LE, Chin KJ. Lumbar neuraxial ultrasound for spinal and epidural anesthesia: A systematic review and meta-analysis. *Reg Anesth Pain Med.* 2016;41(2):251-260.

Tuohy or Quincke needles and risk of intravascular injection during caudal epidural block

58

Why this topic is important

Caudal epidural blocks (CEBs) are widely used for managing lower back pain, radiculopathy, and chronic post-surgery syndromes due to their simplicity and efficacy. However, intravascular injection of local anesthetics during CEBs can lead to severe complications, including systemic toxicity and neurological deficits. Reducing the risk of intravascular injection is a critical safety concern in these procedures.

Needle type is thought to influence the likelihood of intravascular injection, with blunt-tip needles hypothesized to be safer than sharp-tip ones. Yet, limited evidence directly compares the performance of commonly used needles, such as the Tuohy (blunt-tip) and Quincke (sharp-tip) needles, particularly under ultrasound guidance. A recent study by Kim et al. 2024 provides new insights into the role of needle type and procedural factors in minimizing intravascular injection risk during CEBs.

Objectives of this update

- Compare the incidence of intravascular injections using Tuohy and Quincke needles during ultrasound-guided CEBs.

- Identify procedural factors that influence the risk of intravascular injection.

- Provide recommendations for optimizing the safety and efficacy of CEBs.

What is new

The prospective, randomized, controlled study by Kim et al. 2024 involving 230 patients examined the incidence of intravascular injections during ultrasound-guided CEBs with Tuohy and Quincke needles. Key findings include:

- No statistically significant difference in intravascular injection rates between the Tuohy (7.8%) and Quincke needles (13.9%).

- Needle contact with bony structures significantly increased the risk of intravascular injection.

- Anatomical variations in sacral morphology did not influence injection rates.

Detailed findings

Study design

- Population: 230 adults with low back or radicular pain undergoing CEBs were randomized into Tuohy or Quincke needle groups.
- Procedural method: Ultrasound-guided needle placement was followed by digital subtraction angiography (DSA) to detect intravascular injection.

Primary outcomes

1. Intravascular injection rates:
   - Tuohy needle: 7.8% (9/115).
   - Quincke needle: 13.9% (16/115).
   - The difference was not statistically significant, but the practical implications of this difference are worth noting
2. Bony contact and intravascular injection:
   - Bony contact was associated with a significantly higher risk of intravascular injection, highlighting the importance of precise needle positioning.
3. Anatomical variations:
   - Morphological features of the sacrum, including the sacral hiatus angle and diameter, did not affect intravascular injection rates.

Secondary findings

1. Procedure time:
   - Similar across both groups (median: ~ 55 seconds).
2. Pain scores:
   - Both groups reported significant pain relief 30 minutes post-block, with slightly lower scores in the Quincke group.
3. Safety:
   - No cases of dural puncture or neurological sequelae were reported.

Implications for practice

Needle selection and safety

1. Blunt-tip needles:
   - The Tuohy needle did not demonstrate a statistically significant safety advantage over the Quincke needle.
2. Ultrasound guidance:
   - Accurate ultrasound visualization is critical to avoid bony contact and reduce intravascular injection risk.

Procedural considerations

1. Avoid bony contact:
   - Contact with the sacral periosteum can cause vessel injury, emphasizing the importance of precise technique.
2. Fluoroscopy as a supplement:
   - Consider using fluoroscopy in complex cases to confirm needle placement and avoid intravascular injection.

Study limitations and future research

This study had several limitations that should be considered when interpreting the findings. First, the sample size of 230 patients, while calculated for statistical adequacy, may still be insufficient to detect small but clinically relevant differences in intravascular injection rates between needle types. The low number of intravascular injection events (25 out of 230 cases) could have reduced the power to identify statistically significant differences. Additionally, the absence of blinding regarding the needle type for the performing physician introduces the potential for observer bias.

Second, the study monitored pain outcomes only at two time points: before the block and 30 minutes afterward. This limited follow-up might not capture long-term outcomes or complications related to intravascular injection. Variability in patients' analgesic regimens, physical therapy, or subsequent interventions could also confound these results.

Finally, although ultrasound-guided procedures were used, reliance on digital subtraction angiography (DSA) as the gold standard for detecting intravascular injections may not fully replicate real-world clinical settings where DSA is not routinely available.

Further studies are necessary to confirm these findings and explore ways to optimize safety during caudal epidural blocks. Future research should focus on larger, multicenter trials to enhance the generalizability of results. Investigations into additional procedural factors, such as varying angles of needle insertion or alternative needle designs, could provide deeper insights into minimizing intravascular injection risk. Long-term follow-up studies assessing pain relief, patient satisfaction, and potential complications will also be invaluable in refining clinical practice.

Key takeaways

- ☑ Intravascular injection during CEBs is relatively uncommon but remains a significant risk.

- ☑ Bony contact is a critical factor increasing injection risk, regardless of needle type.

- ☑ While Tuohy needles do not significantly reduce injection rates compared to Quincke needles, their blunt design may have advantages in other contexts.

- ☑ Ultrasound guidance is essential for enhancing safety and efficacy in CEBs.

- ☑ Larger, multicenter studies are needed to validate these findings and better understand the impact of needle type and procedural factors on intravascular injection risk.

Additional recommended reading

1. Kim JY, Lee JS, Kim JY, et al. Comparison of the incidence of intravascular injection using the Tuohy and Quincke needles during ultrasound-guided caudal epidural block: A prospective randomized controlled study. *Reg Anesth Pain Med.* 2024;49:17-22.

2. Shin J, Kim YC, Lee SC, et al. A comparison of Quincke and Whitacre needles with respect to risk of intravascular uptake in S1 transforaminal epidural steroid injections: A randomized trial. *Anesth Analg.* 2013;117:1241-7.

3. Park SJ, Yoon KB, Shin DA, et al. Influence of needle-insertion depth on epidural spread and clinical outcomes in caudal epidural injections: A randomized clinical trial. *J Pain Res.* 2018;11:2961 7.

Optimizing spinal anesthesia for ambulatory surgery

59

Why this topic is important

Major ambulatory surgery (MAS) has gained prominence as healthcare systems strive to balance cost-effectiveness and patient satisfaction. Optimizing anesthetic techniques for MAS is crucial as an increasing number of procedures are being performed on an outpatient basis. Spinal anesthesia (SA) has emerged as a viable alternative to general anesthesia (GA), offering distinct advantages such as lower postoperative nausea and vomiting (PONV), reduced opioid use, and faster recovery in selected populations. A recent review by Ledesma et al. 2024 assesses SA's growing role in MAS, highlighting its benefits, limitations, and strategies for overcoming implementation barriers in the outpatient setting.

Objectives of this update

- To evaluate the benefits of spinal anesthesia over general anesthesia in MAS.

- To identify the challenges of implementing SA in outpatient settings.

- To explore strategies for improving its use and mitigating risks.

What is new

Recent evidence highlights the utility of SA for outpatient surgery in reducing complications, improving recovery times, and enhancing patient satisfaction. Short-acting anesthetics like prilocaine and advancements in atraumatic needles have further expanded its safety and feasibility.

Key findings

Advantages of spinal anesthesia in MAS

1. Reduced postoperative complications

   ◦ SA is associated with lower rates of PONV compared to GA, particularly in high-risk populations where systemic sedatives are avoided.

   ◦ It eliminates the need for airway management, reducing the risk of airway-related complications, especially in obese or high-risk patients with conditions like chronic obstructive pulmonary disease (COPD) or obstructive sleep apnea (OSA).

2. Faster recovery

   ◦ Using ultra-short-acting anesthetics (e.g., prilocaine and chloroprocaine) allows quicker motor recovery and ambulation, enabling same-day discharge.

- Studies show earlier discharge times with SA compared to GA in procedures like knee arthroscopy and hernia repairs.

3. Patient comfort and satisfaction

- Patients report higher satisfaction with SA due to fewer side effects like drowsiness or confusion postoperatively.

- When combined with light sedation, SA provides a balanced approach, addressing common patient concerns about remaining awake during surgery.

4. Cost-effectiveness

- SA reduces hospital costs by enabling outpatient procedures and minimizing resource use, including recovery room stays and medications.

Challenges and limitations

1. Technical and procedural barriers

- SA requires precise technique and patient cooperation, which can be challenging in uncooperative patients or those with anatomical variations (e.g., obesity).

- The need for dedicated pre-anesthesia spaces to administer SA before patients enter the operating room can complicate workflows.

2. Post-dural puncture headache (PDPH)

- PDPH remains a concern, with an incidence of up to 5% in younger patients or those undergoing repeated needle attempts. Using atraumatic needles (25-27 gauge) has significantly reduced this risk.

3. Transient neurological symptoms (TNS)

- Although rare, TNS, characterized by sensory alterations or radiating pain, is more frequently reported with lidocaine but is less common with newer agents like prilocaine or bupivacaine.

4. Urinary retention

- Postoperative urinary retention (POUR) is more common with SA than GA, particularly when long-acting anesthetics are used. Strategies like fluid restriction and short-acting drugs can help mitigate this issue.

Practical strategies for implementation

1. Anesthetic selection

- Opt for short-acting local anesthetics like prilocaine to optimize recovery time and minimize complications.

2. Improved patient communication

- Offer light sedation options and clear preoperative explanations of the benefits and process of SA to address patient fears about remaining awake during surgery.

3. Streamlining workflows

- Establish pre-anesthesia rooms to administer SA, reducing OR delays and improving procedural efficiency.

4. Monitoring and prevention

- Use atraumatic needles to lower PDPH risk. Implement protocols to identify and manage POUR proactively, especially in high-risk patients.

Limitations

- Most findings are based on observational studies or single-center trials, limiting generalizability.

- Inconsistent definitions of outcomes like "time to ambulation" make comparisons across studies challenging.

Key takeaways

☑ SA offers significant advantages over GA in MAS, including lower PONV rates, faster recovery, and reduced complications in high-risk populations.

☑ The use of short-acting local anesthetics and atraumatic needles has made SA more feasible and safe for outpatient procedures.

☑ Appropriate protocols and patient selection can mitigate challenges like PDPH, TNS, and POUR.

☑ Further research is essential to optimize its use in MAS and expand its adoption.

Additional recommended reading

1. Ledesma I, Stieger A, Luedi MM, Romero CS. Spinal anesthesia in ambulatory patients: A review of current practices and future directions. *Curr Opin Anaesthesiol.* 2024;37:000-000.

2. Saporito A, Ceppi M, Perren A, et al. Does spinal chloroprocaine pharmacokinetic profile translate into clinical advantages? *J Clin Anesth.* 2019;52:99-104.

3. Stewart J, Gasanova I, Joshi GP. Spinal anesthesia for ambulatory surgery: current controversies and concerns. *Curr Opin Anaesthesiol.* 2020;33:746-752.

Lumbar neuraxial anesthesia in patients with challenging anatomy

60

Why this topic is important

Lumbar neuraxial anesthesia (spinal and epidural) is a cornerstone of anesthesia practice, offering advantages such as improved postoperative outcomes, reduced pulmonary complications, and lower mortality rates than general anesthesia. However, administering these blocks can be technically challenging in patients with altered spinal anatomy due to conditions like scoliosis, degenerative changes, obesity, or prior spinal surgeries. The review by Poots et al. 2024 presents practical strategies, including a detailed examination of the paraspinous (or paramedian) approach, ultrasound-guided techniques, and positioning modifications, to enhance the success and safety of neuraxial blocks in these challenging scenarios.

Objectives of this update

- To highlight the advantages of the paraspinous approach for lumbar neuraxial anesthesia.

- To explore ultrasound-guided techniques for improved accuracy in patients with difficult anatomy.

- To discuss strategies for optimizing needle placement and patient positioning.

What is new

The review by Poots et al. 2024 underscores the value of ultrasound imaging, emphasizing pre-procedural assessments and real-time guidance to improve success rates. It also recommends specific adjustments for unique challenges, such as calcifications, scoliosis, and obesity, which can otherwise hinder traditional approaches.

Key findings

Challenges with midline approaches

- Difficulties with poorly palpable landmarks, narrowed interspinous spaces, and limited lumbar flexion increase the likelihood of bony contact and technical failure.

- Midline techniques in patients with challenging anatomy are associated with higher complication rates, including back pain, post-dural puncture headache, and unsuccessful catheter placement.

Advantages of the paraspinous approach

1. Simplified needle trajectory:

   ◦ The needle is inserted closer to the midline (0.5-1 cm lateral) with a smaller lateral-to-medial angle (5-10°).

   ◦ This technique reduces the range of potential angles required for successful entry into the interlaminar space, making it easier to navigate altered anatomy.

2. Improved tactile feedback:

   ◦ A smoother transition through paraspinal muscles to the ligamentum flavum enhances the ability to detect appropriate structures during insertion.

3. Higher success rates:

   ◦ Randomized controlled trials (RCTs) show significantly better first-attempt success rates with the paraspinous approach than traditional midline techniques.

4. Reduced complications:

   ◦ The paraspinous approach results in lower rates of back pain and post-dural puncture headache.

Role of ultrasound guidance

1. Pre-procedural imaging:

   ◦ Ultrasound aids in identifying spinal landmarks, including the interlaminar spaces and spinous processes, which may be difficult to palpate in obese or elderly patients.

   ◦ The parasagittal oblique (PSO) view provides a qualitative assessment of interlaminar space patency, guiding appropriate needle trajectory.

2. Real-time guidance:

   ◦ Real-time ultrasound-guided techniques are feasible but require expertise. They are particularly beneficial in cases of severe anatomical distortion, though they may increase procedure time.

3. Applications in specific challenges:

   ◦ Obesity: Ultrasound is invaluable for localizing deeper structures and maintaining accuracy during needle advancement.

   ◦ Scoliosis: It helps determine the convex side of the spinal curve, where interlaminar spaces are wider and needle insertion is more likely to succeed.

Specific strategies for challenging scenarios

1. Obesity:

   ◦ To navigate increased tissue resistance, use longer needles (≥ 90 mm) with a stiffer gauge (22 G).

   ◦ Consider the paraspinous approach as a first-line technique due to its higher tolerance for imprecise insertion.

2. Scoliosis:

   ◦ Insert needles on the convex side of the spinal curve to leverage wider interlaminar spaces and minimize the need for medial-to-lateral angulation.

3. Calcification:

   ◦ In patients with calcified spinous processes, adjust the insertion site slightly more lateral (up to 1.5 cm) and increase the lateral-to-medial angle to 15-20°.

4. Targeting L5/S1:

   ◦ The L5/S1 interlaminar space often remains patent in degenerative spinal disease. Ultrasound imaging can help differentiate it from the S1 foramen, ensuring accurate targeting.

DIFFICULT SPINAL ANESTHESIA

Challenges
- **Spinal disease:** Narrow interspinous spaces
- **Obesity:** Soft tissue complicates landmark identification
- **Scoliosis:** Curved spine makes midline access difficult
- **Previous surgery:** Scar tissue complicates access
- **Poor positioning:** Reduces necessary lumbar flexion

Paraspinous approach
- Advantages: Easier needle trajectory, less contact with ligaments, higher success in scoliosis/obesity
- Technique: Insert needle 0.5-1 cm lateral to midline, angled 5°-10° medially
- Benefits: Reduces post-procedure pain and complications such as PDPH.

Paramedian approach
- Advantages: Avoids the need to locate and navigate through the interspinous space
- Technique: Insert needle at a lateral-to-medial angle of 10°-15°
- Benefits: Reduces needle contact with the bony structure, reduces complications and leads to a higher success rate in patients with challenging spinal anatomy

Taylor approach
- Advantages: Useful when other techniques fail and in patients with spinal abnormalities or limited lumbar flexion
- Technique: Insert the needle 1 cm medial to the posterior iliac spine, angled 45°-55° cephalad
- Benefits: Effective alternative, reduces procedure time and patient discomfort

Tailored strategies
- Obese patients: Ultrasound + paraspinous approach + 22G needle to reduce tissue resistance
- Patients with scoliosis: Ultrasound + paraspinous approach
- Patients with degenerative spinal disease: Ultrasound + Taylor approach

Clinical implications

Benefits of the paraspinous approach

- The paraspinous approach simplifies neuraxial block placement, particularly in patients with difficult anatomy, and minimizes the need for repeated needle passes.

- It reduces complications associated with midline approaches, such as back pain and headaches, and improves patient satisfaction.

Integration of ultrasound

- Pre-procedural ultrasound should be considered a routine tool in challenging cases to enhance anatomical visualization and plan needle trajectory.

- Real-time ultrasound may be reserved for complex cases requiring high precision, though it is less practical for routine use.

Recommendations for practice

- Train practitioners in the paraspinous approach and ultrasound-assisted techniques to increase success rates in difficult neuraxial blocks.

- Tailor strategies to individual patient anatomy, leveraging the versatility of ultrasound and alternative approaches.

Limitations

- Most studies cited focus on cadaveric models or non-obese populations, limiting generalizability.

- Evidence for long-term outcomes of ultrasound-guided techniques is sparse.

Key takeaways

- ☑ The paraspinous approach is a valuable alternative to the midline technique for lumbar neuraxial anesthesia in patients with challenging anatomy.

- ☑ Ultrasound imaging enhances procedural success by improving visualization and guiding needle placement.

- ☑ Adapting techniques for specific anatomical challenges, such as obesity, scoliosis, and calcification, improves patient outcomes and reduces complications.

Additional recommended reading

1. Poots C, Chin KJ. Strategies for successful lumbar neuraxial anaesthesia and analgesia in patients with challenging anatomy. *BJA Educ.* 2024;24(2):46—56.

2. Chin KJ, Perlas A, Chan V. The ultrasound-assisted paraspinous approach to lumbar neuraxial blockade: A simplified technique in patients with difficult anatomy. *Acta Anaesthesiol Scand.* 2015;59:668-73.

3. Srinivasan KK, Leo AM, Iohom G, et al. Pre-procedure ultrasound-guided paramedian spinal anaesthesia at L5-S1: Is this better than landmark-guided midline approach? A randomized controlled trial. *Indian J Anaesth.* 2018;62:53-60.

Spinal anesthesia in patients with aortic stenosis

61

Why this topic is important

Aortic stenosis (AS) is a significant challenge for anesthetic management due to the risk of severe hemodynamic instability. Historically, spinal anesthesia (SA) has been considered contraindicated in AS patients, owing to its potential to induce sympathetic blockade and precipitous hypotension. However, there is a lack of robust data to guide clinical practice regarding the safety and efficacy of SA in this high-risk population.

This study by Van Herreweghe et al. 2024 provides critical insights into the hemodynamic effects of SA in patients with moderate or severe AS undergoing lower limb orthopedic surgeries. By evaluating real-world outcomes, it challenges traditional assumptions about the risks associated with SA in AS and explores its viability as an alternative to general anesthesia (GA). These findings are crucial as clinicians strive to balance effective anesthesia with patient safety in this vulnerable group.

Objectives of this update

- To assess SA's safety and hemodynamic impact in patients with moderate or severe AS.

- Examine the perioperative outcomes, including vasopressor use, intensive care unit (ICU) admissions, and mortality.

- To explore the implications of low-dose SA as a potential alternative to GA in managing AS patients.

What is new

This retrospective study by Van Herreweghe et al. 2024 is among the first to provide detailed data on SA in AS patients, addressing its impact on blood pressure stability, need for vasoactive medications, and perioperative outcomes. Key findings include:

1. SA does not significantly increase the risk of intraoperative hemodynamic instability in AS patients.

2. No perioperative cardiac arrests, ICU admissions, or mortality were observed.

3. Low-dose isobaric bupivacaine (10 mg) was well-tolerated, even in severe AS cases.

Key findings

Study design

- Participants: 35 patients with AS (16 moderate and 19 severe) undergoing lower limb orthopedic surgery under SA between 2017 and 2022.

- Anesthetic protocol: SA was performed at < L2 with 10 mg of isobaric bupivacaine 0.5%.

- Outcomes: Blood pressure stability (mean arterial pressure [MAP]), vasopressor use, ICU admissions, and 30-day mortality.

Results

1. Hemodynamic stability:

   - Absolute MAP values fell below 65 mmHg in 11% of total readings, with no significant difference between moderate (7%) and severe (13%) AS groups.
   - Relative MAP reductions > 20% from baseline occurred in 27% of readings, slightly higher in severe AS patients (33%) but not statistically significant.

2. Vasoactive interventions:

   - 23% of patients required vasoactive drugs intraoperatively, including norepinephrine (9%), phenylephrine (17%), and ephedrine (14%).
   - No cases required prolonged vasopressor therapy or aggressive hemodynamic resuscitation.

3. Perioperative outcomes:

   - No ICU admissions, cardiac arrests, or deaths occurred within 24 hours or 30 days postoperatively.
   - All patients completed surgery without conversion to GA.

Clinical implications

Reassessing spinal anesthesia in AS patients

- Safety profile: The findings suggest that SA, when performed with low-dose isobaric bupivacaine, is a safe option for AS patients undergoing lower limb surgery, challenging traditional contraindications.

- Hemodynamic management: While relative hypotension was observed in some cases, these episodes were manageable with standard vasoactive interventions and did not result in adverse outcomes.

- Practical application: SA may offer advantages over GA by avoiding the risks associated with intubation and systemic anesthesia in AS patients.

Tailored anesthetic approaches

- Low-dose technique: The use of isobaric bupivacaine at reduced doses appears to minimize sympathetic blockade, preserving hemodynamic stability.

- Patient selection: Careful preoperative evaluation and planning remain essential, with SA reserved for selected AS patients undergoing non-cardiac surgery.

Limitations and future directions

Study limitations

- Small sample size: The study included only 35 patients, limiting the generalizability of its findings.

- Retrospective design: Lack of randomization and potential for selection bias must be considered when interpreting results.

Future research

- Conduct prospective, multicenter trials to validate the safety of SA in AS patients across diverse surgical settings.

- Explore alternative dosing and baricity of local anesthetics to optimize outcomes further.

- Investigate long-term outcomes, including recovery trajectories and chronic pain management in AS patients receiving SA.

Key takeaways

☑ Low-dose isobaric spinal anesthesia appears safe and effective for patients with moderate or severe aortic stenosis undergoing lower limb surgery.

☑ Hemodynamic stability was maintained, and hypotensive episodes were manageable with standard vasoactive interventions.

☑ No perioperative cardiac arrests, ICU admissions, or mortality were observed, supporting the use of SA as an alternative to general anesthesia in selected cases.

Additional recommended reading

1. Van Herreweghe I, De Fré O, Polus F, et al. Spinal anesthesia in patients with aortic stenosis: A research report. *Reg Anesth Pain Med.* 2024;0:1-3.

2. Johansson S, Lind MN. Central regional anesthesia in patients with aortic stenosis: A systematic review. *Dan Med J.* 2017;64:A5407.

3. Nishimura RA, Otto CM, Bonow RO, et al. AHA/ACC guideline for the management of patients with valvular heart disease. *Circulation.* 2014;129:2440-92.

Multimodal pain management and outcomes

Regional anesthesia
for pain in ICU patients

62

Why this topic is important

Pain management is a cornerstone of intensive care, with up to 50% of ICU patients experiencing moderate-to-severe pain during their stay. Uncontrolled pain can prolong mechanical ventilation, delay recovery, and lead to complications such as post-traumatic stress disorder (PTSD) and delirium. While systemic opioids remain a primary strategy, they come with risks like respiratory depression, sedation, and gastrointestinal dysfunction.

Regional anesthesia (RA) has emerged as a valuable tool for ICU pain management, offering targeted analgesia with fewer systemic side effects. Recent advances in ultrasound-guided techniques and the development of novel blocks have expanded the indications for RA in critical care settings. This update summarizes the finding of a recent review by Campbell et al. that explores how RA can be effectively integrated into ICU pain management to improve outcomes.

Objectives of this update

- To summarize the applications of regional anesthesia in ICU settings.

- To evaluate the benefits of RA in reducing ICU length of stay (LOS), ventilator days, and opioid consumption.

- To address barriers to the adoption of RA in critical care.

What is new

A recent review by Campbell et 2024 highlights innovative uses of RA in managing complex ICU conditions like cerebral vasospasm and ventricular storm. It also emphasizes ultrasound-guided advancements that make these techniques safer and more accessible for critically ill patients.

Applications of regional anesthesia in critical care

Abdominal and thoracic blocks

- Thoracic epidural anesthesia (TEA): Traditionally used for thoracoabdominal pain, TEA improves respiratory outcomes, reduces cardiac stress, and decreases ICU LOS. However, its use is limited by risks such as epidural hematoma and hypotension, particularly in anticoagulated patients.

- Erector spinae plane block (ESPB): A safer alternative to TEA, ESPB provides effective thoracoabdominal analgesia without the risks associated with neuraxial techniques. It supports early extubation and mobilization in patients with rib fractures, pancreatitis, or thoracic surgery.

- Quadratus lumborum (QL) and transversus abdominis plane (TAP) blocks: These blocks are effective for abdominal wall pain and are increasingly used for surgeries like laparotomy and hysterectomy. QL blocks may offer visceral analgesia, making them suitable for more complex abdominal procedures.

Head and neck blocks

- Stellate ganglion block (SGB): Emerging as a treatment for refractory cerebral vasospasm and ventricular dysrhythmias, SGB may reduce ICU admissions and improve survival in select populations. Its utility extends to post-craniotomy pain management, where monitoring mental status is critical.

Upper and lower extremity blocks

- Brachial plexus blocks: Effective for upper limb surgeries and trauma, these blocks reduce opioid use and improve tissue perfusion in conditions like replantation surgery.

- Motor-sparing blocks (e.g., PENG block): These newer techniques provide analgesia without compromising motor function, facilitating early ambulation and rehabilitation for lower limb injuries.

Benefits of regional anesthesia in critical care

1. Reduced ICU length of stay

   ◦ Studies report significant reductions in ICU and hospital LOS with RA compared to systemic opioids, particularly in thoracic and abdominal procedures.

2. Decreased opioid consumption

   ◦ RA minimizes opioid requirements, reducing side effects like respiratory depression and ileus. For example, ESPB has been shown to lower postoperative opioid use by up to 50% in cardiac and thoracic surgery patients.

3. Improved functional recovery

   ◦ RA enables earlier extubation, ambulation,

and participation in physical therapy, accelerating recovery and reducing complications like deep vein thrombosis (DVT).

4. Potential mortality benefits

   ◦ RA's role in managing life-threatening conditions such as ventricular storm and cerebral vasospasm may improve survival in critically ill patients.

Barriers to adoption

1. Resource limitations

   ◦ The lack of trained personnel, ultrasound equipment, and standardized protocols limits the widespread use of RA in ICUs.

2. Complexity in critically ill patients

   ◦ Challenges like altered anatomy, anti-coagulation, and difficulty in assessing pain levels in sedated patients complicate block placement.

3. Limited awareness and training

   ◦ Many ICU providers need to become more familiar with RA techniques, highlighting the need for multidisciplinary education and collaboration.

Future directions

Expanding research and education

- More randomized controlled trials are needed to validate the benefits of RA in ICU populations and establish clear guidelines.

- Educational initiatives targeting intensivists and ICU staff can bridge knowledge gaps and promote interdisciplinary care.

Leveraging technology

- Adopting advanced ultrasound-guided techniques and real-time monitoring tools can enhance the safety and efficacy of RA in critical care.

Key takeaways

- ☑ Regional anesthesia offers targeted pain relief, reducing opioid use and improving recovery in critically ill patients.

- ☑ Novel applications, such as managing cerebral vasospasm and ventricular storm, highlight RA's expanding role in ICU care.

- ☑ Education, technology, and standardized protocols can address barriers like resource limitations and lack of training.

- ☑ Continued research is essential to optimize RA applications and ensure safety in ICU populations.

Additional recommended reading

1. Campbell A, Jacoby M, Hernandez N. Critical care innovations: navigating pain relief in intensive care - the role of regional anesthesia. *Curr Opin Anaesthesiol*. 2024;37(5):547-552.

2. Chin KJ, El-Boghdadly K. Mechanisms of action of the erector spinae plane (ESP) block: a narrative review. *Can J Anaesth*. 2021;68:387-408.

3. Greene JJ, Chao S, Tsui BCH. Clinical outcomes of erector spinae plane block for midline sternotomy in cardiac surgery: a systematic review and meta-analysis. *J Cardiothorac Vasc Anesth*. 2024;38:964-973.

Multimodal pain management and opioid use in shoulder arthroplasties

63

Why this topic is important

Shoulder arthroplasties, including total, reverse, and partial replacements, have grown significantly due to advancements in surgical techniques and implant designs. As painful procedures with a high demand for effective postoperative pain control, they highlight the necessity of optimizing analgesic strategies. Multimodal pain management, which combines opioids with additional analgesic modes (e.g., NSAIDs, acetaminophen, or nerve blocks), offers the potential to improve outcomes by reducing opioid use and associated complications.

A recent population-based by Liu et al. 2024 provides valuable insights into the effectiveness of multimodal pain management in both inpatient and outpatient settings, analyzing its association with opioid utilization, postoperative recovery, and healthcare costs.

Objectives of this update

- To examine the impact of multimodal pain management on opioid consumption in inpatient and outpatient shoulder arthroplasties.

- To evaluate its influence on outcomes like length of stay (LOS), costs, and opioid-related complications.

- To determine how adding nerve blocks modifies the effects of multimodal pain strategies.

What is new

The study by Liu et al. 2024, which utilized data from over 176,000 shoulder arthroplasties performed between 2010 and 2019, is one of the largest analyses of multimodal pain management for shoulder surgery. It highlights the differing effects of multimodal strategies in inpatient versus outpatient settings and emphasizes the role of nerve blocks in improving outcomes.

Key findings

Study population

- Sample size: 176,225 procedures: 169,679 inpatient and 6,546 outpatient shoulder arthroplasties.

- Utilization of multimodal analgesia:
  - 75.7% of inpatient cases utilized multimodal analgesia, with the most common regimen being opioids combined with one additional mode (34.5%).
  - Only 37.8% of outpatient cases incorporated multimodal analgesia, reflecting room for improvement in outpatient pain protocols.

Opioid utilization

- Inpatient setting:
  - Multimodal analgesia with > 2 additional modes (excluding nerve blocks) reduced postoperative day 1 opioid consumption by 19.4%.
  - Opioid utilization was reduced by 6.0% for the entire hospital stay.
  - The addition of nerve blocks further amplified reductions in opioid use.
- Outpatient setting:
  - Surprisingly, multimodal analgesia was associated with a 13.7% increase in opioid utilization, possibly due to increased use in higher-risk patients or insufficient integration of non-opioid modes.

Other outcomes

- Length of stay (LOS) and costs:
  - Inpatients showed minimal or no reductions in LOS or hospital costs with multimodal analgesia.
  - Outpatients experienced increased costs with multimodal strategies, reflecting the complexity of managing pain in ambulatory settings.
- Opioid-related adverse events:
  - No significant reduction in naloxone administration (a marker for opioid-related complications) was observed in either setting, indicating opportunities for further optimizing multimodal regimens.

Clinical implications

Tailoring multimodal strategies

- In the inpatient setting, combining > 2 additional analgesic modes with nerve blocks significantly reduces opioid consumption, supporting their use in multimodal protocols.
- For outpatients, the observed increase in opioid utilization suggests a need for better integration of multimodal strategies, particularly through expanded use of nerve blocks and non-opioid analgesics.

Addressing gaps in care

- Only 37.8% of outpatient shoulder arthroplasties employed multimodal analgesia, highlighting an area for improvement in outpatient pain management practices.
- Standardized protocols emphasizing the early incorporation of multimodal techniques and nerve blocks could enhance outcomes in both settings.

Practical recommendations

- Prioritize nerve blocks as part of multimodal regimens to maximize opioid-sparing benefits, especially for inpatients.
- Optimize outpatient multimodal strategies by addressing barriers such as time constraints, patient education, and resource availability.

Limitations

- Retrospective design limits the ability to establish causal relationships.
- The outpatient subgroup had a smaller sample size, potentially impacting the generalizability of findings.
- Data on pain scores and patient satisfaction were unavailable, which could provide a more comprehensive view of multimodal analgesia's effectiveness.

Key takeaways

☑ Multimodal analgesia reduces inpatient opioid use, particularly when combined with nerve blocks, but has mixed results in outpatient settings.

☑ Greater adoption of multimodal strategies in outpatient care is needed to improve outcomes.

☑ Further research is necessary to optimize multimodal pain management protocols and address gaps in outpatient analgesic practices.

Additional recommended reading

1. Liu H, Zhong H, Zubizarreta N, et al. Multimodal pain management and postoperative outcomes in inpatient and outpatient shoulder arthroplasties: A population-based study. *Reg Anesth Pain Med.* 2024;49:1-12.

2. Memtsoudis SG, Poeran J, Cozowicz C, et al. Impact of multimodal analgesia on outcomes in orthopedic surgery: A population-based study. *Anesthesiology.* 2018;129(4):689-699.

3. Soffin EM, YaDeau JT. Enhanced recovery after surgery for primary hip and knee arthroplasty: A review of the evidence. *Br J Anaesth.* 2016;117(suppl 3):iii62-iii72.

Regional anesthesia and persistent opioid use and chronic pain after noncardiac surgery

64

Why this topic is important

Chronic postsurgical pain (CPSP) and persistent opioid use are significant concerns after surgery, with implications for patient quality of life and public health. Opioid-related issues, including dependence and overdose, have become critical societal challenges, prompting the exploration of strategies to minimize opioid exposure. Regional anesthesia (RA) is a cornerstone of multimodal analgesia, reducing acute postoperative pain and opioid consumption. However, its long-term benefits for reducing CPSP and prolonged opioid use remain uncertain. A recent systematic review and meta-analysis[1] address these questions, offering valuable insights for perioperative pain management.

Objectives of this update

- To evaluate whether RA reduces the risk of prolonged opioid use following elective noncardiac surgeries.

- To assess the role of RA in decreasing the incidence of CPSP.

- To provide evidence-based recommendations for integrating RA into clinical practice to improve postoperative outcomes.

What is new

This comprehensive analysis by Pepper et al. 2024 synthesizes data from 37 randomized controlled trials (RCTs) and is the first to assess the relationship between RA and prolonged opioid use. It highlights a potential role for RA in reducing both persistent opioid use and CPSP, particularly within the first six months postoperatively.

Key findings

Study design and methodology

- Population: 4948 adult patients undergoing elective noncardiac surgery, analyzed across 37 RCTs.

- Interventions: Various RA techniques, including epidurals, nerve blocks (femoral, paravertebral, transversus abdominis plane), and field blocks (e.g., serratus plane).

- Primary outcomes:

  ◦ Persistent opioid use (opioid consumption ≥2 months post-surgery).

  ◦ CPSP (pain ≥3 months post-surgery).

Results

1. Prolonged opioid use

   ◦ Regional anesthesia reduced the likelihood of prolonged opioid use by 52%, with an absolute risk reduction of 14%.

2. Chronic postsurgical pain (CPSP)

   ◦ CPSP rates were significantly reduced at three and six months, but no differences were observed at 12 months

3. Acute pain and opioid use

   ◦ Pain scores and opioid use were lower in the first 24-48 hours with regional anesthesia, but differences were not significant by 72 hours.

4. Adverse events

   ◦ Regional anesthesia showed similar rates of adverse events to control groups, with a slight increase in hypotension associated with neuraxial blocks.

Clinical implications

Reducing opioid use and chronic pain

- Prolonged opioid use: RA may lower the incidence of persistent opioid use by improving early pain control and reducing the need for discharge opioid prescriptions.

- CPSP: RA potentially mitigates the transition from acute to chronic pain by interrupting central sensitization processes.

Practical recommendations

- Include RA as part of multimodal analgesia for patients at high risk of CPSP or opioid dependence.

- Prioritize RA for surgeries associated with significant postoperative pain or known risks of chronic pain (e.g., thoracotomies, mastectomies).

Limitations to consider

- Heterogeneity of techniques: Variability in RA methods and surgical procedures limits generalizability.

- Short-term follow-up: Most benefits were observed within six months, with limited data on long-term effects.

Future research directions

1. Surgery-specific analyses: Evaluate RA's efficacy in specific surgical populations and high-risk procedures.

2. Long-term studies: Assess the impact of RA on opioid use and CPSP beyond 12 months.

3. Mechanistic studies: Investigate how RA interrupts neuroplastic changes associated with chronic pain.

Key takeaways

☑ RA reduces prolonged opioid use and CPSP at 3 and 6 months after surgery.

☑ No significant effect was observed on CPSP at 12 months, suggesting the need for extended research.

☑ RA improves acute pain outcomes and is a vital component of opioid-sparing analgesic strategies.

Additional recommended reading

1. Pepper CG, Mikhaeil JS, Khan JS. Perioperative regional anesthesia on persistent opioid use and chronic pain after noncardiac surgery: A systematic review and meta-analysis of randomized controlled trials. *Anesth Analg.* 2024;139:711-22.

2. Weinstein EJ, Levene JL, Cohen MS, et al. Local anesthetics and regional anesthesia versus conventional analgesia for preventing persistent postoperative pain in adults and children. *Cochrane Database Syst Rev.* 2018;4:CD007105.

3. Harkouk H, Fletcher D, Martinez V. Paravertebral block for the prevention of chronic postsurgical pain after breast cancer surgery. *Reg Anesth Pain Med.* 2021;46:251-257.

Emerging insights and comparisons of techniques

Single injection or continuous interscalene block for shoulder surgery analgesia

65

Why this topic is important

Major shoulder surgeries, such as arthroplasty and rotator cuff repair, often cause significant postoperative pain. Regional anesthesia, specifically the interscalene brachial plexus block (ISBPB), is widely used to manage this pain. Traditionally, continuous local anesthetic infusions have been favored over single injections for their longer-lasting effects. However, recent advances in multimodal analgesia regimens, which incorporate non-opioid medications like dexamethasone and ketorolac, may alter the balance between the two methods. A recent study by Rhyner et al. 2024 evaluates whether a continuous infusion offers superior analgesia to a single bolus of local anesthetic when both are used within a comprehensive multimodal analgesia strategy.

Objectives of this update

- To assess whether a continuous infusion improves pain management compared to a single injection in ISBPB for shoulder surgery.

- To evaluate the opioid-sparing effects of each method.

- To determine if functional recovery and patient satisfaction differ between techniques.

What is new

- The study by Rhyner et al. (2024) is among the first to compare single-injection and continuous-infusion ISBPB techniques in the context of multimodal analgesia, challenging assumptions about the necessity of continuous catheters in this setting.

Key findings

Study design

- Participants: 60 patients undergoing elective shoulder arthroplasty or rotator cuff repair.

- Intervention groups:

  - Single-injection group: 20 mL of 0.5% ropivacaine, with the catheter removed post-bolus.

  - Continuous-infusion group: 20 mL of 0.5% ropivacaine followed by a continuous infusion of 0.2% ropivacaine (6-8 mL/hour) for 48 hours.

- Primary outcome: Cumulative intravenous morphine consumption at 24 hours post-surgery.

- Secondary outcomes: Pain scores, functional outcomes, and adverse events over 48 hours.

Results

1. Opioid consumption:

   - Morphine use at 24 hours was similar: 10 mg (continuous infusion) vs. 14 mg (single injection), with no significant difference.

   - No differences were observed at 12, 36, or 48 hours post-surgery.

2. Pain scores:

   - Pain scores at rest and during movement were comparable between groups throughout the 48-hour period.

3. Functional outcomes:

   - Shoulder range of motion and patient satisfaction scores were similar across groups.

4. Adverse events:

   - Both techniques had low complication rates, and no persistent nerve deficits or neuropathic pain were reported.

Clinical implications

Impact on analgesic choice

- Single injection sufficiency: The findings suggest that a single-injection ISBPB, when combined with multimodal analgesia (e.g., acetaminophen, NSAIDs, and adjuncts like dexamethasone), is as effective as a continuous infusion, potentially eliminating the need for catheter placement.

- Reduced resource demands: Avoiding continuous infusions eliminates the logistical challenges of catheter management, such as dislodgement risk and the need for acute pain service follow-up.

Recommendations for practice

- Prioritize single-injection ISBPB for shoulder surgeries when multimodal analgesia is administered, particularly in outpatient settings.

- Consider continuous infusion only for patients with complex pain needs, such as chronic pain syndromes or high opioid tolerance.

Limitations

- The trial was unblinded, introducing potential performance bias.

- Findings may not generalize to patients undergoing ambulatory shoulder surgeries, where prolonged analgesia could be more valuable.

Key takeaways

☑ Single-injection ISBPB provides equivalent pain control and opioid-sparing benefits compared to continuous infusion when used with multimodal analgesia.

☑ Continuous infusions may no longer be necessary for most patients, simplifying postoperative management.

☑ These findings support shifting clinical practice toward single-injection ISBPB, particularly for routine shoulder surgeries.

Additional recommended reading

1. Rhyner P, Cachemaille M, Goetti P, et al. Single-bolus injection of local anesthetic, with or without continuous infusion, for interscalene brachial plexus block in the setting of multimodal analgesia: A randomized controlled unblinded trial. *Reg Anesth Pain Med.* 2024;49:313-319.

2. Fredrickson MJ, Ball CM, Dalgleish AJ. Analgesic efficacy of ropivacaine 0.2% for interscalene brachial plexus block in shoulder surgery. *Reg Anesth Pain Med.* 2008;33:114-119.

3. Abdallah FW, Brull R. Is continuous peripheral nerve block needed for outpatient orthopedic surgery? *Anesth Analg.* 2017;124:1036-1038.

Faster onset of block with lidocaine-bupivacaine mixture in ultrasound-guided SCBPs

66

Why this topic is important

Effective anesthesia for upper limb surgeries relies on a combination of rapid onset, complete conduction blockade (CCB), and prolonged postoperative analgesia. Ultrasound-guided supraclavicular brachial plexus blocks (SCBPBs) have revolutionized this field by offering precision with lower anesthetic volumes (fig-1).

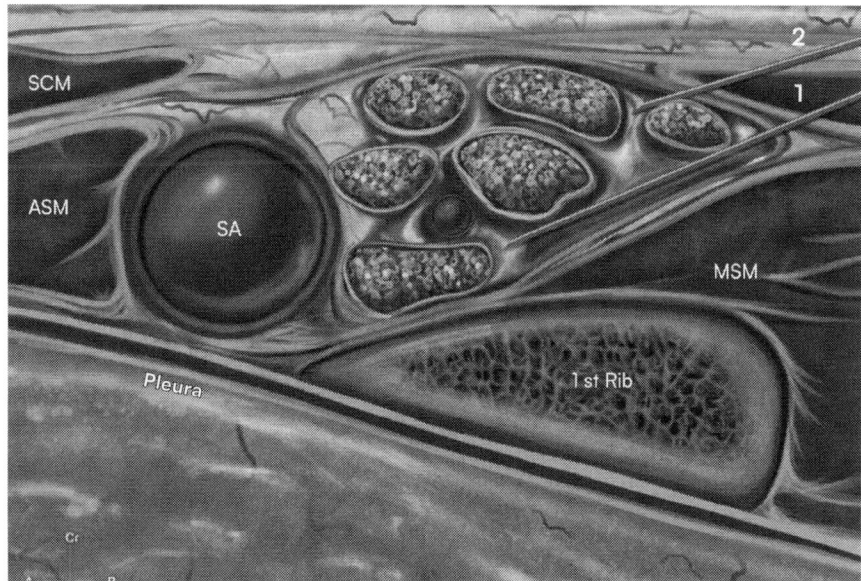

Fig-1. Supraclavicular brachial plexus block; Reverse ultrasound anatomy with needle insertion in-plane. SA, Subclavian artery; MSM, Middle scalene muscle; SCM, sternocleidomastoid muscle; ASM, anterior scalene muscle. Image taken from NYSORA LMS. https://nysoralms.com/

A recent study by Sripriya et al. 2024 evaluates whether mixing lidocaine (for rapid onset) with bupivacaine (for prolonged duration) provides significant clinical benefits over bupivacaine alone, potentially optimizing SCBPBs for faster surgical readiness and effective pain management.

Objectives of this update

- To compare the time to CCB between lidocaine-bupivacaine mixture and bupivacaine alone.

- To assess the duration of postoperative analgesia and block effectiveness across nerve territories.

- To explore the implications of anesthetic mixtures for clinical practice in low-volume SCBPBs.

What is new

The study by Sripriya et al. 2024 establishes that a lidocaine-bupivacaine mixture significantly reduces the time to CCB and improves block consistency compared to bupivacaine alone, providing a balanced solution for faster onset and adequate postoperative pain control.

Key findings

Study design

- Participants: 63 patients undergoing upper extremity surgeries under SCBPB.

- Groups:

  - Group L: 20 mL of 2% lidocaine with epinephrine.

  - Group B: 20 mL of 0.5% bupivacaine.

  - Group LB: 20 mL of equal parts 2% lidocaine with epinephrine and 0.5% bupivacaine.

- Primary outcome: Time to CCB (total composite score [TCS] of 16/16).

- Secondary outcomes: Duration of postoperative analgesia, sensory-motor block assessment, and safety outcomes.

Results

1. Time to CCB:

   - Group LB achieved CCB faster (16 ± 7 min) than Group B (21 ± 7 min), with a comparable onset to Group L (14 ± 6 min).

   - The proportion of patients attaining CCB within 40 minutes was highest in groups L and LB (95%) compared to group B (48%).

2. Postoperative analgesia:

   - Median analgesia duration was the longest in Group B (12.2 hours), followed by Group LB (8.3 hours) and Group L.

3. Nerve territory differences:

   - Proximal nerve blockade (musculocutaneous, radial) occurred faster than distal nerves (median, ulnar) across all groups, with Group B showing significant delays.

4. Safety:

   - No complications, such as persistent neurological deficits or adverse events, were reported in any group.

Clinical implications

Benefits of lidocaine-bupivacaine mixture

- Rapid onset: The mixture significantly reduces time to CCB, optimizing surgical readiness for fast-paced operating environments.

- Balanced analgesia: While slightly shorter than bupivacaine alone, the mixture provides sufficient postoperative pain relief for many surgical procedures.

Practical considerations

- Tailored use: The mixture is ideal for cases requiring quick onset and adequate analgesia duration, such as ambulatory or same-day discharge procedures.

- Dose precision: Using 20 mL volumes ensures safety while maximizing efficiency in achieving nerve blockade.

Limitations and future directions

- The study's 40-minute observation limit may have underestimated the full potential of bupivacaine in achieving CCB.

- Findings are specific to upper extremity bone surgeries, limiting generalizability to other procedures.

Key takeaways

☑ A 20 mL mixture of lidocaine and bupivacaine achieves a faster onset of CCB than bupivacaine alone while providing longer postoperative analgesia than lidocaine alone.

☑ This combination is particularly suited for low-volume ultrasound-guided SCBPBs in time-sensitive surgical settings.

☑ These findings support integrating anesthetic mixtures into routine clinical practice for improved efficiency and patient outcomes.

Additional recommended reading

1. Sripriya R, Sivashanmugam T, Rajadurai D, Parthasarathy S. Equal mixture of 2% lidocaine with adrenaline and 0.5% bupivacaine 20 mL provided faster onset of complete conduction blockade during ultrasound-guided supraclavicular brachial plexus block than 20 mL of 0.5% bupivacaine alone: A randomized double-blind clinical trial. *Reg Anesth Pain Med.* 2024;49:104-109.

2. Laur JJ, Bayman EO, Foldes PJ, et al. Mixing lidocaine and bupivacaine for brachial plexus block: A randomized trial. *Reg Anesth Pain Med.* 2012;37:28-33.

3. Cuvillon P, Nouvellon E, Ripart J, et al. Pharmacodynamics of lidocaine and bupivacaine mixtures in peripheral nerve blocks. *Anesth Analg.* 2009;108:641-649.

Reducing catheter migration: ISAFE technique for adductor canal blocks

67

Why this topic is important

Continuous adductor canal block (ACB) catheters have become key in managing postoperative pain for total knee arthroplasty (TKA), providing effective analgesia while preserving quadriceps strength. This allows for early ambulation, quicker recovery, and potentially reduced hospital stay. However, one persistent issue is catheter migration, which can compromise analgesic efficacy and necessitate interventions. A recent study by Gleicher et al. 2024 evaluates the interfascial plane between the sartorius muscle and femoral artery (ISAFE) technique, a novel approach hypothesized to reduce catheter migration, against the conventional insertion method.

Objectives of this update

- To assess the comparative rates of catheter migration with ISAFE and conventional ACB placement techniques.

- To explore the implications of migration rates on pain scores, opioid use, and clinical outcomes.

- To provide insights into how improving catheter placement can enhance recovery after TKA.

What is new

- This controlled trial by Gleicher et al. 2024 demonstrates that the ISAFE technique significantly reduces catheter migration rates. It underscores the technique's importance in determining block reliability and influencing pain management and patient outcomes.

Findings on catheter migration and clinical outcomes

Methodology

This study enrolled 97 patients undergoing TKA. Participants were randomly assigned to two groups:

1. ISAFE group: Catheters were placed in the fascial plane between the sartorius muscle and femoral artery, ensuring greater tip stability.

2. Conventional group: Catheters were placed lateral to the femoral artery adjacent to the saphenous nerve.

The catheter position was assessed via ultrasound 24 hours postoperatively to determine migration. Pain scores, opioid consumption, and sensory block coverage were evaluated on postoperative days (POD) 1 and 2.

Key results

Migration rates

- ISAFE technique: Only 18.6% of catheters migrated outside the adductor canal.

- Conventional technique: Migration occurred in 44.9% of catheters.

The reduced migration rate in the ISAFE group supports its ability to maintain catheter placement within the intended anatomical plane, which is critical for effective analgesia.

Pain scores

- Resting pain scores were significantly lower in the ISAFE group:

  - POD 1 median score: 1.0 vs. 3.0 in the conventional group.

  - Similar findings were reported on POD 2.

- Pain during movement and opioid consumption did not differ significantly between groups, though trends favored the ISAFE technique.

Proximity to the saphenous nerve

- ISAFE catheters remained closer to the saphenous nerve, enhancing block efficacy for deep and superficial sensory targets.

Catheter stability

- Migration distances were shorter in the ISAFE group, with better tip retention within the adductor canal.

- No significant differences in skin fixation site stability were observed between groups.

Clinical implications

ISAFE technique advantages

The ISAFE approach tunnels the catheter tip more securely within the adductor canal, reducing migration risks. This has the following clinical benefits:

- Improved pain management: Reduced migration ensures consistent analgesic coverage, particularly for deep tissue structures contributing significantly to TKA-related pain.

- Enhanced recovery: Reliable analgesia supports early mobilization, a critical component of fast-track recovery protocols.

- Decreased interventions: Lower migration rates may reduce the need for catheter repositioning, saving time and resources.

Impact on recovery pathways

Optimizing catheter placement can enhance the efficacy of multimodal pain management strategies. With the ISAFE technique, patients are more likely to achieve effective pain relief with fewer complications, facilitating earlier discharge and improved patient satisfaction.

Limitations

- Follow-up duration: Assessments were limited to the first 48 hours postoperatively. Migration rates and pain outcomes beyond this period remain unknown.

- Sample size: While adequately powered for the primary outcome, a larger cohort could provide greater insight into secondary endpoints.

- Generalizability: Findings may vary across institutions, patient populations, and surgical protocols.

Key takeaways

☑ The ISAFE technique significantly reduces catheter migration compared to the conventional approach.

☑ Improved stability results in lower pain scores at rest during the first 48 hours postoperatively.

☑ Reliable catheter placement enhances overall analgesic efficacy, supporting faster recovery and reduced resource utilization.

☑ Future studies should focus on long-term outcomes and broader applications of the ISAFE technique.

Additional recommended reading

1. Gleicher Y, dos Santos Fernandes H, Peacock S, et al. Comparison of migration rates between traditional and tunneled adductor canal block catheters: a randomized controlled trial. *Reg Anesth Pain Med.* 2024;49:423-428.

2. Dos Santos Fernandes H, Siddiqui N, Peacock S, et al. Interfascial space between sartorius muscle and femoral artery (ISAFE): a suggested approach for adductor canal catheter placement. *J Clin Anesth.* 2022;76:110571.

3. Fujino T, Yoshida T, Kawagoe I, et al. Migration rate of proximal adductor canal block catheters placed parallel versus perpendicular to the nerve after total knee arthroplasty: a randomized controlled study. *Reg Anesth Pain Med.* 2023;48:420-424.

Intraoperative landmark-based genicular nerve block or periarticular infiltration in TKA

68

Why this topic is important

Postoperative pain control after total knee arthroplasty (TKA) remains a critical aspect of patient recovery. Effective pain management improves early mobility, reduces hospital stays, and minimizes complications such as opioid dependence. With a growing emphasis on opioid-sparing techniques, multimodal analgesia combining regional anesthesia with peripheral nerve blocks has become the standard of care. Two commonly used techniques are periarticular infiltration (PAI) and genicular nerve block (GNB), both of which aim to provide motor-sparing analgesia. This update explores the findings of a recent randomized controlled trial comparing intraoperative landmark-based GNB with PAI, with a focus on their roles in postoperative pain management in TKA patients.

As new techniques emerge, it is vital to understand their practical implications for improving patient outcomes while mitigating the risks of motor blockade and excessive opioid use. The study of Kertkiatkachorn et al. 2024 aims to clarify their relative benefits and limitations in clinical practice by delving into their efficacy[1].

Objectives of this update

- To compare the pain relief efficacy of GNB and PAI in patients undergoing TKA.

- To analyze the differences in pain control at rest versus movement between these two techniques.

- To assess secondary outcomes such as opioid consumption, time to first rescue analgesia and functional recovery.

- To discuss potential risks and complications, including motor blockades and sleep disturbances.

- To make informed decisions on when to use GNB or PAI based on clinical factors.

What is new

The randomized trial by Kertkiatkachorn et al. 2024 compared two widely adopted techniques-GNB and PAI-used in TKA within a multimodal analgesic framework. It broke new ground by analyzing the efficacy of intraoperative landmark-based GNB against the more established PAI, particularly when combined with continuous adductor canal block (CACB). While both techniques are proven to be effective for static pain relief, the study highlights key differences in pain control during movement, opioid consumption, and functional recovery-factors critical in guiding perioperative decisions for TKA patients.

Overview of analgesic techniques

1. Periarticular Infiltration (PAI):

PAI involves injecting a mixture of local anesthetics, nonsteroidal anti-inflammatory drugs (NSAIDs), and epinephrine directly into the tissues surrounding the knee joint (fig-1). The surgeon performs this technique intraoperatively and targets multiple structures, including the collateral ligaments, capsule, and periarticular tissues. PAI is favored for its simplicity, motor-sparing benefits, and effectiveness when combined with peripheral nerve blocks such as the adductor canal block (ACB).

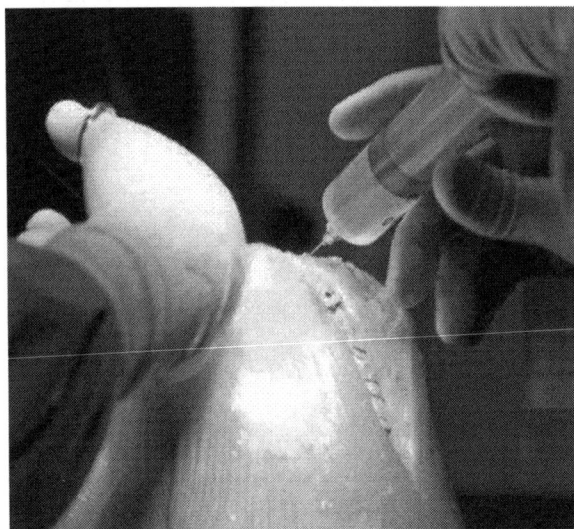

Fig-1. Periarticular infiltration of local anesthetics for total knee arthroplasty (TKA).
Image taken from NYSORA LMS. https://nysoralms.com/

2. Genicular Nerve Block (GNB):

GNB, a newer technique, aims to anesthetize the terminal branches of the femoral, sciatic, and obturator nerves that innervate the knee joint (fig-2). It can be performed intraoperatively using anatomical landmarks rather than ultrasound, making it convenient for surgeons during TKA. By targeting specific genicular nerves (superior medial, inferior medial, superior lateral, and sometimes inferior lateral), GNB provides localized pain relief with fewer needle insertions, reducing the risks associated with higher-volume infiltration techniques.

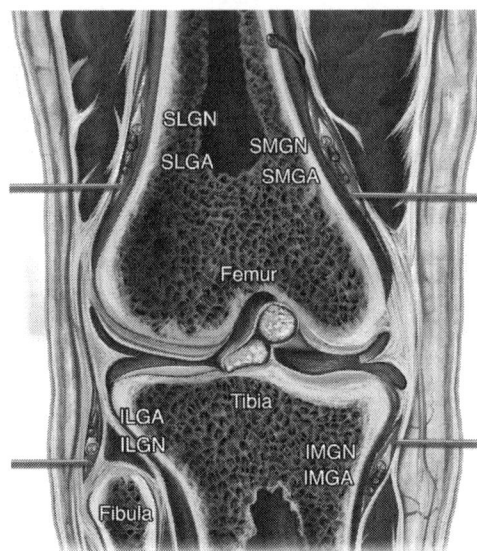

Fig-2. Local anesthetic spread around the superolateral genicular nerve (SLGN), the superomedial genicular nerve (SMGN), the inferolateral genicular nerve (IMGN), and the inferomedial genicular nerve (IMGN). Image taken from NYSORA LMS. https://nysoralms.com/

Study findings and comparative analysis

Primary outcome: Pain scores at 12 hours postoperatively

- Resting pain: Both PAI and GNB were highly effective at controlling resting pain at 12 hours postoperatively, with median pain scores of 0 in both groups. The difference between groups was negligible, with a median difference of 0 and a confidence interval well within the non-inferiority margin. This demonstrates that GNB is just as effective as PAI for pain relief at rest.

- Pain during movement: Movement-related pain is a significant concern in the early postoperative period because it impacts a patient's ability to mobilize and rehabilitate. The PAI group showed superior pain control during movement, with a median pain score of 1.5 compared to 2 in the GNB group. GNB failed to demonstrate non-inferiority for movement-related pain, with a median difference of 0.9, which crossed the predefined non-inferiority margin of 1. This suggests that PAI may offer better dynamic pain control in the early postoperative period.

Opioid consumption and time to rescue analgesia

- Opioid consumption: One of the critical goals of modern multimodal analgesia is to reduce reliance on opioids, which can lead to adverse side effects and complications like nausea, sedation, and respiratory depression. In this trial, the PAI group consumed significantly less intravenous morphine within the first 12 hours postoperatively. The median opioid consumption in the PAI group was 0 mg (range 0-0), while the GNB group had a slightly higher consumption (0 mg, range 0-4). However, by 24 and 48 hours, opioid consumption between the two groups was comparable.

- Time to first rescue analgesia: The time to first rescue analgesia (i.e., the time until the patient required additional pain medication) was notably longer in the PAI group (15.7 hours) compared to the GNB group (7.4 hours). This suggests that PAI provides longer-lasting pain relief in the immediate postoperative period, which may reduce the need for early opioid intervention.

Functional recovery and motor blockade

- Functional performance: The trial measured functional recovery using the timed-up-and-go (TUG) test and the Knee Society Knee Score (KSKS). Patients in the PAI group demonstrated better functional recovery, with significantly faster TUG test results on postoperative days (POD) 1 and 2. This could be attributed to better movement-related pain control in the PAI group.

- Motor blockade: One concern with PAI is the risk of inadvertent motor blockade, particularly of the tibial and common peroneal nerves. In this study, partial motor blockade was more frequent in the PAI group than in the GNB group. This suggests that GNB may be a safer option for minimizing motor blockade, especially in patients where motor preservation is crucial for early mobilization.

Sleep disturbance and other complications

- Sleep disturbance: On postoperative day 0, patients who received GNB reported higher incidences of sleep disturbance compared to those in the PAI group. Sleep is an important factor in recovery, and poor pain control can lead to interrupted sleep, delayed healing, and prolonged hospital stays. The higher incidence of sleep disturbance in the GNB group may reflect less effective dynamic pain control in the early postoperative hours.

- Adverse events: Both techniques were generally well-tolerated, with no serious adverse events reported. However, the study highlights the need for cautious dosing of local anesthetics during PAI to avoid excessive infiltration, which could contribute to motor blockade or local anesthetic toxicity.

Comparison of periarticular infiltration and genicular nerve block in total knee arthroplasty.

Parameter	Periarticular Infiltration (PAI)	Genicular Nerve Block (GNB)
Pain control (Rest)	Effective (Non-inferior to GNB)	Effective (Non-inferior to PAI)
Pain control (movement)	Superior for movement-related pain	Inferior for dynamic pain
Opioid consumption (12 hrs)	Lower opioid consumption	Higher opioid consumption
Motorsparing	Risk of partial motor blockade	Lower risk of motor blockade
Functional recovery (TUG test)	Faster recovery (better TUG results)	Slower recovery
Complexity of procedure	Simple, performed by a surgeon	Fewer injections, motor-sparing

Practical considerations

When to use PAI

- Better for dynamic pain relief: PAI provides superior pain relief during movement, making it ideal for patients where early mobilization is critical, such as those undergoing aggressive postoperative rehabilitation.

- Simple and efficient: The surgeon performs PAI directly during surgery, offering a streamlined process that can be easily integrated into routine TKA procedures. This is particularly beneficial in high-volume surgical centers where time efficiency is important.

- Motor-sparing but risk of blockade: While generally motor-sparing, PAI has a slightly higher risk of causing partial motor blockades, particularly in the tibial and common peroneal nerves. Careful attention to infiltration sites and volumes is required.

When to use GNB

- Less invasive and fewer needle insertions: GNB requires fewer needle insertions compared to PAI, potentially reducing the risk of local anesthetic toxicity and complications related to high-volume infiltrations.

- Motor-sparing advantage: GNB may be a better option for patients where preserving motor function is a high priority, particularly in cases where extensive peripheral nerve blocks or high anesthetic volumes have already been used.

- Inferior for movement-related pain: Despite its advantages, GNB does not provide the same level of dynamic pain relief as PAI. It may be less suitable for patients expected to engage in early postoperative mobilization.

Key takeaways

☑ PAI provides superior movement-related pain control, with longer-lasting analgesia and reduced early opioid consumption compared to GNB.

☑ GNB offers a motor-sparing advantage with fewer needle insertions, making it useful in patients where motor preservation is crucial.

☑ Functional recovery is faster with PAI, as demonstrated by better TUG test results on POD 1 and 2.

☑ Sleep disturbances were more common in patients who received GNB, likely due to inferior dynamic pain control.

☑ The choice of technique should be patient-specific, balancing factors like early mobility, opioid use, and the risk of motor blockades.

Additional recommended reading

1. Kertkiatkachorn W, Ngarmukos S, Tanavalee A, et al. Intraoperative landmark-based genicular nerve block versus periarticular infiltration for postoperative analgesia in total knee arthroplasty: A randomized non-inferiority trial. *Reg Anesth Pain Med.* 2024;49:669-676.

2. Teng Y, Jiang J, Chen S, et al. Periarticular multimodal drug injection in total knee arthroplasty. *Knee Surg Sports Traumatol Arthrosc.* 2014;22:1949-57.

3. Albrecht E, Guyen O, Jacot-Guillarmod A, et al. The analgesic efficacy of local infiltration analgesia vs femoral nerve block after total knee arthroplasty: A systematic review and meta-analysis. *Br J Anaesth.* 2016;116:597-609.

Single-injection intertransverse process block or PVB at T2 level

69

Why this topic is important

Thoracic pain management often necessitates precise regional anesthesia techniques to provide effective analgesia while minimizing risks. The paravertebral block (PVB) is a well-established thoracic and upper extremity pain method, including sympathetically maintained pain conditions such as complex regional pain syndrome (CRPS). The PVB achieves analgesia by targeting the thoracic sympathetic chain and adjacent nerve structures (fig-1). However, its proximity to critical structures like the pleura and intercostal vessels increases the risk of complications such as pneumothorax and neurovascular injury.

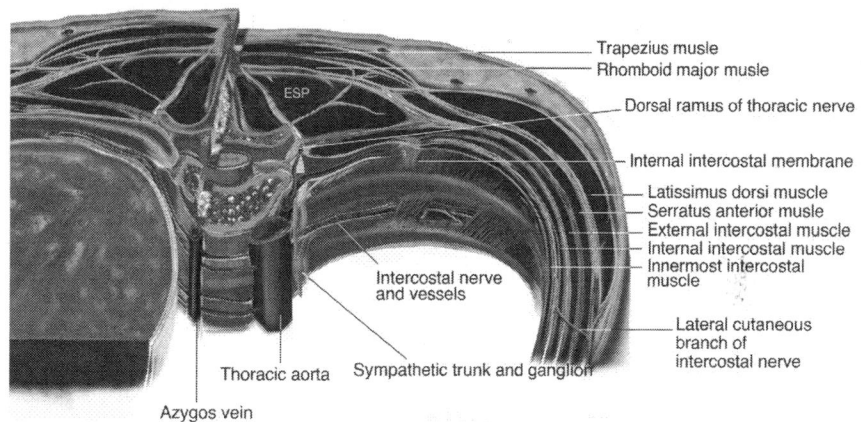

Fig-1. Anatomy of the paravertebral space. ESP, erector spinae muscles.
Image taken from NYSORA LMS. https://nysoralms.com/

The intertransverse process (ITP) block, a recently developed technique, offers a potentially safer alternative by positioning the needle further from the pleura. Despite its safety advantages, there is limited data on whether the ITP block provides nerve coverage comparable to the PVB. A study by Kim et al. 2024 evaluates and compares these two blocks' injectate spread and nerve coverage at the T2 level using cadaveric models, shedding light on their relative efficacy and potential clinical applications.

Objectives of this update

- To compare the efficacy of PV and ITP blocks in achieving sympathetic chain coverage at the T2 level.

- To analyze the anatomical spread of injectate and its implications for thoracic and upper extremity pain management.

- To assess the relative safety profiles of the two techniques regarding pleural and nerve involvement.

What is new

This is the first cadaveric study to directly compare the spread and nerve staining achieved by single-injection ITP and PVBs at the T2 vertebral level. The findings reveal differences in sympathetic chain coverage, dorsal and ventral ramus involvement, and potential safety advantages of the ITP block.

Study findings

Methodology

- Study design: Cadaveric study using 16 soft-embalmed cadavers.

- Intervention: Ultrasound-guided single-injection PV and ITP blocks were performed on opposite sides of each cadaver. Each block used 10 mL of dye solution.

- Assessment: Dissection was conducted to evaluate dye spread and staining of key anatomical structures, including:

  ○ The thoracic sympathetic chain at the T2 level.

  ○ Dorsal and ventral rami.

  ○ Dorsal root ganglion (DRG).

Results

1. Sympathetic chain coverage

   ○ PVB consistently stained the T2 sympathetic ganglion in all 16 cadavers (100%).

   ○ ITP block provided sympathetic ganglion staining in 68.8% of cases, indicating less reliable sympathetic chain coverage.

2. Dorsal and ventral rami

   ○ The ITP block achieved superior staining of the dorsal ramus (93.8%) compared to the PVB (68.8%).

   ○ Ventral ramus staining was slightly higher with the PVB (93.8%) than the ITP block (81.3%).

3. Dorsal root ganglion (DRG)

   ○ DRG staining was observed in 75% of ITP blocks compared to 50% of PVBs, suggesting a potential advantage for ITP blocks in targeting conditions involving the DRG.

4. Safety considerations

   ○ ITP block positions the needle further from the pleura and major vascular structures, potentially reducing the risk of pneumothorax and neurovascular injury.

Comparison of PVB vs. ITP block.

Criteria	PB block	ITP block
Sympathetic chain coverage	100% consistent at T2 level	68.8% consistent
Dorsal rami coverage	68.8%	93.8%
Dorsal root ganglion coverage	50%	75%
Ventral rami coverage	93.8%	81.3%
Clinical applications	Sympathetically maintained pain	Posterior thoracic pain
Risks	Pneumothorax, vascular injury	Lower risk of pleural puncture

Clinical implications

Role of the PVB

The PVB remains the gold standard for addressing sympathetically maintained thoracic wall pain and conditions requiring reliable sympathetic chain coverage. Its superior ability to stain the sympathetic ganglion makes it highly effective for CRPS and post-thoracotomy pain syndromes. However, its proximity to the pleura and intercostal vessels necessitates careful technique to minimize risks such as pneumothorax or bleeding.

Role of the ITP block

- The ITP block is less reliable for sympathetic chain coverage but demonstrates superior dorsal ramus and DRG staining. This suggests a potential role in treating dorsal rami-mediated pain, such as myofascial pain syndromes or thoracic radiculopathies.

- The block's safer anatomical positioning makes it a promising option for patients at higher risk of pleural or vascular complications, such as those with preexisting pulmonary disease or anticoagulation therapy.

Choosing between techniques

The target nerves and specific clinical indications should guide the choice between PV and ITP blocks:

- PVB is preferred for comprehensive, sympathetic chain coverage.

- ITP block may be advantageous when dorsal ramus or DRG involvement is the primary goal or when safety concerns preclude PVB use.

Limitations

- Cadaveric model: The soft-embalmed cadavers used may not replicate the dynamics of live tissues, such as tissue elasticity and blood flow, which can influence injectate spread.

- Single injectate volume: The study only used 10 mL of dye solution, which may not reflect real-world clinical practice where varying volumes are employed based on patient anatomy and clinical goals.

- Focus on T2 level: Findings are specific to the T2 vertebral level and may not generalize to other thoracic levels.

Key takeaways

☑ PVB consistently and comprehensively covers the thoracic sympathetic chain, making it the standard for sympathetically maintained pain and thoracic wall analgesia.

☑ ITP block achieves superior dorsal ramus and DRG staining, suggesting potential applications for dorsal rami-mediated pain and thoracic radiculopathies.

☑ The safer needle positioning of the ITP block reduces the risk of complications such as pneumothorax, making it a viable alternative for high-risk patients.

☑ Further refinement of ITP block techniques and additional research are needed to enhance its consistency and expand its clinical applications.

Additional recommended reading

1. Kim JY, Lee UY, Kim DH, et al. Comparison of injectate spread and nerve coverage between single-injection intertransverse process block and paravertebral block at the T2 level: A cadaveric study. *Reg Anesth Pain Med.* 2024;49:436-439.

2. Karmakar MK. Thoracic paravertebral block. *Anesthesiology.* 2001;95:771-80.

3. Cho TH, Kwon HJ, O J, et al. The pathway of injectate spread during thoracic intertransverse process (ITP) block: Micro-CT findings and anatomical evaluations. *J Clin Anesth.* 2022;77:110646.

Medial and between-transverse-process approaches to ESPB

70

Why this topic is important

The erector spinae plane block (ESPB) is an increasingly utilized regional anesthesia technique first introduced for thoracic neuropathic pain management and later applied to postoperative pain control across a range of thoracic and abdominal surgeries. Its benefits include providing targeted analgesia while reducing the need for systemic opioids, minimizing side effects, and promoting faster recovery. However, there is considerable variability in the injectate spread and clinical effectiveness of ESPB's largely due to differences in needle placement and approach.

The lack of consensus on optimal injection sites has led to varied outcomes in clinical practice, with reports of limited anterior spread that may reduce the ESP block's effectiveness, particularly in procedures requiring broad or anterior coverage. A recent anatomical study[1] compares two ESPB techniques- the medial transverse process (MED) approach and the between transverse processes (BTWN) approach-to assess which provides greater spread and, potentially, enhanced analgesic coverage. By better understanding how each technique impacts the spread to relevant nerve structures, clinicians can make informed decisions to improve patient outcomes.

Objectives of this update

- Determine injectate spread patterns: Evaluate and compare the spread of injectate between the MED and BTWN ESP block techniques in human cadavers.

- Understand clinical implications: Identify the practical impacts of each approach on analgesic coverage, particularly for procedures requiring broader or deeper reach.

- Assist in technique selection: Guide practitioners in selecting the most appropriate ESP block approach based on anatomical spread patterns and intended clinical outcomes.

What is new

- Enhanced anterior and epidural spread with BTWN: BTWN ESP blocks showed greater anterior and epidural spread, suggesting improved effectiveness for pain relief in thoracic surgeries that affect both anterior and posterior structures.

- Limited anterior spread in MED: MED ESP blocks were more confined to posterior structures, indicating limited reach to anterior thoracic targets and potentially reduced analgesic efficacy for certain procedures.

- Differential neural involvement: BTWN consistently stained both dorsal and ventral rami, dorsal root ganglion (DRG), and in some cases, provided intrathecal spread, indicating broader neural involvement compared to MED.

Clinical study overview

Methods

In the study by Harbell et al. 2024, researchers used 14 unembalmed human cadavers divided into two groups of seven. Each cadaver received a single 20 mL injection of methylene blue dye at either the MED or BTWN injection site at T4-T5. MED injections were administered at the medial transverse process, while BTWN injections were administered between the transverse processes. Following injection, anatomical dissections documented dye spread in three planes-cephalocaudal (vertical), mediolateral (horizontal), and anterior-posterior-and assessed its reach to specific neural structures such as dorsal and ventral rami, DRG, and epidural spaces.

Results

1. Cephalocaudal spread:

   ○ MED: Dye spread cephalocaudally from C4-T12 in most cases but tended to stay within the thoracic region, showing less consistency in reaching upper cervical or lower lumbar regions.

   ○ BTWN: BTWN injections demonstrated broader and more reliable cephalocaudal spread, with dye typically extending from C5-T11. The increased vertical spread suggests BTWN's potential for more extensive analgesic coverage across multiple thoracic levels.

2. Mediolateral spread:

   ○ MED: Medial injections showed limited lateral spread, reaching the iliocostalis muscle in only five cases. This confinement to posterior structures indicates that MED may be best suited for superficial thoracic pain management.

   ○ BTWN: BTWN injections consistently extended laterally to the iliocostalis muscle in all cadavers, offering more consistent lateral coverage that could improve efficacy in procedures involving extensive lateral and posterior structures.

3. Anterior spread and neural structure staining:

   ○ MED: Dye reached the dorsal rami in all MED injections, but ventral rami and DRG staining was inconsistent, occurring in only a subset of cases. Limited reach to these anterior structures suggests MED's reduced efficacy in conditions requiring broad paravertebral or anterior nerve coverage.

   ○ BTWN: BTWN achieved reliable dorsal and ventral rami staining in nearly all cases, with significant DRG involvement. This consistent anterior spread supports BTWN as the preferred approach for procedures where anterior thoracic pain control is essential, such as thoracotomies or cardiac surgeries.

4. Epidural spread:

   ○ MED: MED injections demonstrated minimal epidural spread (median of one spinal level), suggesting limited central neuraxial involvement and reduced efficacy for cases where central analgesic reach is desired.

   ○ BTWN: The BTWN approach showed more extensive epidural spread, ranging from 3 to 12 spinal levels (median: 5 levels). Some injections even demonstrated contralateral and intrathecal spread, indicating BTWN's capacity to achieve broader central analgesic coverage, which is beneficial for more complex surgeries.

Discussion

Anatomical spread and clinical implications

1. Enhanced anterior and epidural reach with BTWN: The BTWN approach showed superior anterior spread, reaching critical anterior structures like the ventral rami and dorsal root ganglion (DRG). This broader spread aligns with the clinical needs of patients undergoing thoracic surgeries, such as thoracotomies or mastectomies, that affect both anterior and posterior areas. Additionally, BTWN's extensive epidural spread supports its use in cases requiring broad central coverage, as seen in bilateral thoracic or complex cardiac

procedures. Its ability to achieve consistent anterior spread enhances its potential as a comprehensive analgesic approach.

2. MED's confinement to posterior structures: In contrast, MED ESP blocks were confined largely to posterior structures, with limited reach to paravertebral spaces, ventral rami, or epidural areas. While MED may be sufficient for localized posterior thoracic pain, its restricted spread may limit its effectiveness for procedures involving the anterior thoracic region or central neuraxial requirements. The MED approach may be best suited to superficial thoracic surgeries where deep analgesic spread is unnecessary.

3. Clinical relevance for neuropathic thoracic pain: Given that the BTWN approach achieved consistent staining of both dorsal and ventral rami, it may be especially useful in managing thoracic neuropathic pain or other cases where the involvement of anterior nerve structures is required. This broader neural reach could translate to better pain control in complex neuropathic conditions or cases where standard ESP blocks have been less effective.

Practical considerations for ESP block selection

1. Technique implications:

   ○ MED approach: MED ESP blocks are technically simpler, with the needle contacting the medial transverse process, which may limit the spread to posterior structures. This technique could be favorable in settings where broad anterior spread is not necessary or where simpler, quicker administration is beneficial.

   ○ BTWN approach: By targeting the intertransverse tissue complex (ITTC) anterior to the transverse processes, BTWN ESP blocks avoid direct bony contact, allowing injectate to spread through fascial planes and reach broader anterior regions. This approach may, however, require greater technical expertise and careful positioning to ensure effective reach without intrathecal injection risk.

2. Clinical recommendations:

   ○ For superficial or localized thoracic surgeries, the MED approach provides targeted posterior coverage, meeting analgesic needs with minimal central or anterior reach. .

   ○ For broad thoracic and anterior abdominal procedures, the BTWN approach offers more extensive analgesic coverage, benefiting patients who require extended paravertebral or epidural spread for complex, multi-level thoracic or neuropathic pain control.

Comparative anatomy of MED vs. BTWN ESPB spread.

Parameter	MED ESP Block	BTWN ESP Block
Cephalocaudal spread	C4-T12 (variable, confined to thoracic)	C5-T11 (more consistent spread)
Mediolateral spread	Limited, occasional iliocostalis reach	Consistent to iliocostalis muscle
Anterior structure reach	Primarily dorsal rami	Dorsal and ventral rami, DRG
Epidural spread	0-3 levels (median: 1)	3-12 levels (median: 5), occasional contralateral
Ideal clinical use	Superficial thoracic analgesia	Broad thoracic and abdominal analgesia

Key takeaways

☑ Broader analgesic coverage with BTWN: The BTWN approach demonstrated superior anterior and epidural spread, making it suitable for thoracic and anterior abdominal procedures requiring extensive analgesic coverage.

☑ Targeted analgesia with MED: MED ESP blocks were largely confined to posterior muscle layers, with limited anterior or epidural reach, indicating suitability for localized posterior thoracic analgesia.

☑ Enhanced utility for neuropathic pain with BTWN: Consistent reach to ventral and dorsal rami suggests BTWN may be advantageous for patients with complex neuropathic thoracic pain.

☑ Decision-making for technique selection: Clinicians should consider the BTWN ESP block for enhanced anterior spread, especially in cases requiring broad analgesic reach, while the MED ESP block may suit cases requiring minimal central effects.

Additional recommended reading

1. Harbell, M. W., Langley, N. R., Seamans, D. P., et al. "Evaluating two approaches to the erector spinae plane block: an anatomical study." *Reg Anesth Pain Med* 2024;48:495-500.

2. Forero, M., Adhikary, S. D., Lopez, H., et al. "The erector spinae plane block: a novel analgesic technique in thoracic neuropathic pain." *Reg Anesth Pain Med* 2016;41:621-7.

3. Diwan, S., Garud, R., Nair, A. "Thoracic paravertebral and erector spinae plane block: a cadaveric study demonstrating different site of injections and similar destinations." *Saudi J Anaesth* 2019;13:399-401.

Single-injection and multiple-injection intertransverse process blocks

71

Why this topic is important

Regional anesthesia techniques for truncal blocks continue to evolve, with the intertransverse process (ITP) block gaining attention as a promising alternative to paravertebral and erector spinae plane (ESP) blocks. The ITP block is commonly used for managing thoracic wall pain in surgeries but has variations in technique-specifically, single-injection versus multiple-injection methods.

The choice between these techniques impacts the block's efficacy, ease of application, and safety. Understanding their relative effectiveness is critical for optimizing clinical practices and minimizing procedural invasiveness. A recent trial by Nielsen et al. 2024 provides the first direct comparison of single-injection and multiple-injection ITP blocks, assessing their ability to anesthetize thoracic dermatomes and their potential clinical applications.

Objectives of this update

- To compare the effectiveness of single-injection versus multiple-injection ITP blocks in anesthetizing thoracic dermatomes.

- To evaluate secondary outcomes, including sensory coverage, thermographic changes, and hemodynamic effects.

- To explore the potential of these techniques for broader clinical applications.

What is new

- This is the first randomized, non-inferiority, crossover trial to evaluate the single-injection ITP block compared to the multiple-injection technique, demonstrating that single-injection is non-inferior in dermatome coverage.

Key findings

Study design and participants

- Participants: 12 healthy male volunteers.

- Design: Randomized, blinded, crossover trial with each participant receiving both techniques in separate sessions.

- Techniques:

  ○ Single-injection: 21 mL of ropivacaine 7.5 mg/mL at the T4/T5 level with sham injections at T2 and T6.

  ○ Multiple-injection: 7 mL of ropivacaine 7.5 mg/mL at T2/T3, T4/T5, and T6/T7 levels.

- Primary outcome: Number of anesthetized thoracic dermatomes.

- Secondary outcomes: Sensory mapping (cm²), thermography results, mean arterial pressure (MAP) changes, and block application satisfaction.

Results

1. Dermatome coverage

   ○ The mean difference in anesthetized thoracic dermatomes between single-injection and multiple-injection techniques was 0.82, indicating non-inferiority of the single-injection technique.

   ○ Both techniques showed variable sensory blockade of the ipsilateral thoracic wall, with no clinically significant differences.

2. Sensory mapping

   ○ Combined anterior and posterior cutaneous block areas were larger with the multiple-injection technique, but this difference was not statistically significant.

   ○ Posterior sensory coverage was significantly greater in the multiple-injection group.

3. Thermographic analysis

   ○ No significant differences in temperature changes were observed between techniques.

○ Both techniques showed statistically significant thermographic changes at various thoracic levels and time points compared to the baseline, supporting the block's efficacy.

4. Hemodynamic effects

   ○ MAP decreased in the multiple-injection group at 30 and 60 minutes post-block, likely due to sympathetic trunk blockade. However, these changes were clinically insignificant.

5. Block application satisfaction

   ○ Pain scores during needle placement were similar between techniques, though sham injections in the single-injection group resulted in slightly lower scores at non-injection sites (e.g., T2 and T6).

Clinical implications

Benefits of single-injection ITP block

- Non-inferior efficacy: Provides comparable dermatome coverage to the multiple-injection technique, simplifying the procedure.

- Reduced invasiveness: Requires fewer injections, minimizing patient discomfort and potential complications.

- Time efficiency: Faster to perform, particularly beneficial in high-volume clinical settings.

Considerations for multiple-injection ITP block

- Enhanced sensory coverage may be preferable for surgeries requiring broader posterior thoracic wall analgesia.

- Hemodynamic monitoring: The potential for MAP changes necessitates careful patient selection and intraoperative monitoring.

Limitations

- A small sample size limits generalizability.

- The volunteer population may not reflect the response in surgical patients with altered physiology.

- Lack of data on block duration and long-term outcomes.

Key takeaways

☑ Single-injection ITP block is non-inferior to multiple-injection in anesthetizing thoracic dermatomes, offering a simpler, less invasive option.

☑ Both techniques provide effective ipsilateral thoracic wall coverage with variable posterior sensory involvement.

☑ Further studies are needed to explore the clinical utility of ITP blocks in diverse surgical settings.

Additional recommended reading

1. Nielsen MV, Tanggaard K, Bojesen S, et al. Efficacy of the intertransverse process block: single or multiple injection? A randomized, non-inferiority, blinded, crossover trial in healthy volunteers. *Reg Anesth Pain Med.* 2024;49:708-715.

2. Uppal V, Sondekoppam RV, Sodhi P, et al. Single-injection versus multiple-injection technique of ultrasound-guided paravertebral blocks: a randomized controlled study comparing dermatomal spread. *Reg Anesth Pain Med.* 2017;42:575-81.

3. Zhang H, Qu Z, Miao Y, et al. Comparison between ultrasound-guided multi-injection intertransverse process and thoracic paravertebral blocks for major breast cancer surgery: A randomized non-inferiority trial. *Reg Anesth Pain Med.* 2023;48:161-6.

Made in the USA
Middletown, DE
11 June 2025

76843155R00192